the
HEART LIVES
by BREAKING

A Grandmother's Observations
of Two Sons with Children
Born with Tay-Sachs Disease

GAY LORD

THE HEART LIVES BY BREAKING
*A Grandmother's Observations of Two Sons
with Children Born with Tay-Sachs Disease*

Book title is from "The Testing Tree" by Stanley Kunitz, published in "Collected Poems," Norton & Compnay, 2000.

Published by
GDP Press
Westwood, Massachusetts

ISBN: 978-0-578-47126-6

Library of Congress Cataloging-in-Publication Data is available.

9 8 7 6 5 4 3 2 1

Cover and interior design by www.DominiDragoone.com
Printed in the United States of America

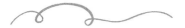

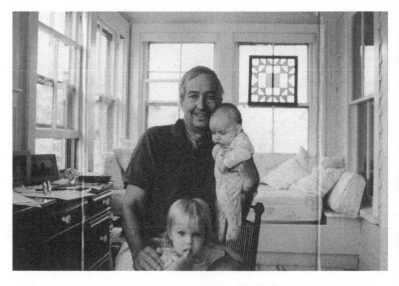

Charles P. Lord holding Hayden,
with his hand on Taylor's shoulder

FOR CHARLES PILLSBURY LORD

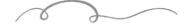

those mottoes stamped on his name-tag:
conscience, ambition, and all that caring
—STANLEY KUNITZ, "THE LONG BOAT"

CONTENTS

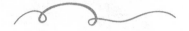

NEW LIVES..1

FIRST YEAR, FIRST BIRTHDAY 7

A DIAGNOSIS 14

STILL NO ANSWERS 20

NEWS THAT ONLY COMES TO OTHERS.....................26

A CHRISTENING AND A THANKSGIVING....................32

COPING..38

TELLING TAYLOR 46

CHRISTMAS 1999 51

HAYDEN AND CAMERON:
    THE SAME DISEASE, UNIQUE BABIES.....................59

TWO BIRTHDAYS..66

SPRING 2000...71

TAYLOR AT THREE...78

HAYDEN HAS A BABY SISTER...................................84

SEPTEMBER 2000: NEW YORK AND GREEN-WOOD.......91

NOVEMBER 2000: CHANGES;
    ANOTHER THANKSGIVING...................................97

HAYDEN: BEFORE CHRISTMAS, 2000.................... 105

PEACEFUL SORROW:
    "HEAVEN LIES ABOUT US IN OUR INFANCY".......... 111

FAREWELL AT GREEN-WOOD, CHRISTMAS 2000........ 119

JANUARY 2001... 126

FEBRUARY 2001: TAYLOR, CAMERON,
    A NEW BABY-AND BELLS!................................ 133

ALIVE IN THE DARK TIME...................................... 140

MAY 4, 2001.. 144

SAYING GOODBYE: CAMERON'S LAST WEEK............. 149

MAY 19, 2001: TO CALL MYSELF BELOVED 157

GATHERED AT GREENWOOD FOR CAMERON............ 167

AFTERWORD.. 172

ABOUT THE AUTHOR... 175

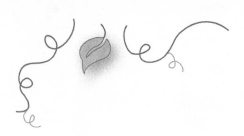

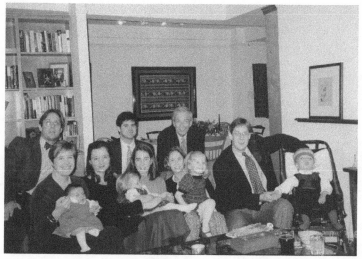

Front Row: Alison holding Annie, Blyth, Deirdre holding Cameron, Gay holding Taylor, Tim holding Hayden's hand. Back Row: Charlie, Miko, Grandfather Charlie.

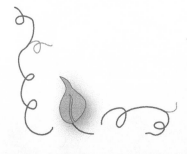

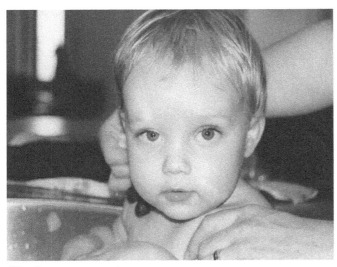

Hayden

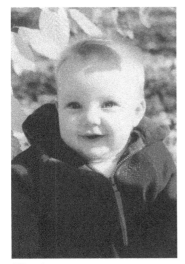

Hayden

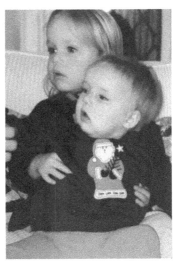

Taylor and Hayden

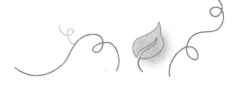

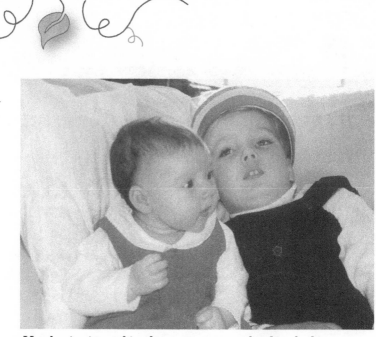

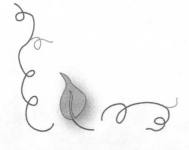

*Hayden is pictured in the crown presented to him by his nurse
Benga—who has conferred on him an honorary chiefdom.
Hayden is Chief Maiyegun of Ekuru, honored "for an act
of courage, sacrifice, and most of all endurance, making the
world a better place to dwell." Maiyegun is a Yoruba word
that means "individual who brightens the world by his act."
That is the Hayden we love and cherish.*

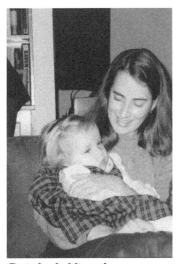

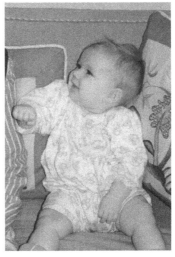

Deirdre holding sleepy
Cameron

Cameron

Taylor and Cameron
at bedtime

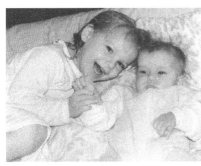

Taylor and Cameron

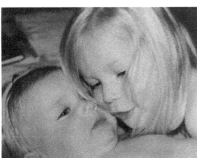

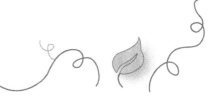

1

NEW LIVES

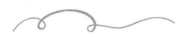

MY SLEEPLESSNESS AND POUNDING HEART IN JANUARY AND February of 1997 were not caused by fear or anxiety. It had never occurred to me to be frightened about birth—not even when anticipating the delivery of twins in a dingy hospital in the tropical heat of Panama City, the Republic of Panama. Now, however, tremors of anticipation ran through me and waves of excited questions crossed my mind.

We were waiting for our first grandchild to be born to Charlie, one of our twins, and his wife Blyth Taylor Lord. I lay awake imagining the joys of grandparenthood, wondering whether "we" would have a boy or a girl, how soon we would be able to visit and to hold the new baby, and what "she" would call us when she began to talk. I thought about where the baby would sleep in the house in Washington and in the cottage in Nantucket. Would her parents want to use the bassinet made for me out of a laundry basket in 1935, the year I was born?

I fantasized about these small things and about the aspects of the world I would be able to share with the new child. I replayed memories of my relationship with my paternal grandmother, Lala, and my maternal grandfather, Grampy. Would this child read aloud to me in my older age as I had to Lala? Would this boy or girl hear from Charlie the recounting of fiercely held principles, as I had from Grampy—my head bowed under the weight of his heavy, gentle hand?

The 3:00 a.m. hours were filled with these thoughts. There was nothing fearful about these musings; in fact, these were joyful, if wakeful, midnight hours. On February 8, 1997, a few of these questions were answered.

Taylor Myers Lord, a baby girl, was born on this day at 2:30 a.m. in Brigham and Womens' Hospital in Boston. Grandfather Charlie and I were on a train on our way to New York to see a performance to be given by young people who had been trained by our actor son, Tim, who is the identical twin of the new baby's father.

We learned of the birth when the boys' younger sister, Deirdre, boarded the train in Wilmington. She stood in the doorway of the car where we were sitting and excitedly delivered a brief message: "The baby wait is over. It's a girl, and her name is Taylor!"

It was always a short stop in Wilmington, and there was little time to talk as Deirdre had spent several minutes finding our location in the train. It had been a long delivery, but we learned that Blyth and the little girl were well, and the new father was ecstatic. We had a glass of bad train wine with our lunch to celebrate the new arrival.

The next day, we went to church at St. Bartholomew's, thinking of all the people, present and absent, who would care deeply about this birth. In my letter to Taylor, written when she was a day old, I was able pass on something we heard that morning, perfect words for someone so new to this world: "May the bright morning star rise in your heart."

My journal entries for the following week, February 9th to 15th, mentioned feelings of anticipation and the need for self control. We longed to be in Boston but thought we should give the new parents time to adjust and also try not to intrude on the time that Blyth's parents would have in the first week after the birth, for the baby was also the first grandchild in the Taylor family.

A week later, a taxi deposited us in front of the tiny half-house in Cambridge. I rushed ahead of grandfather Charlie and up the front steps to find our son Charlie in the tiny entry at the bottom of the steep staircase up to the apartment. Barely taking the time to give my son a kiss of love and congratulations, I called out over his shoulder: "Where is she?" Somehow, I'd had visions of him in the entry hall carrying the baby in his arms, something which was not possible given the fact that the temperature was 4 degrees below zero that day. Everyone remembers my abrupt and enthusiastic entry into Taylor's life.

What a beautiful baby she was! We stayed in Cambridge for a few days and were so entranced that we even watched her sleep, sometimes on the ample bosom of a lovely woman who came for two weeks to help, but mostly blanketed warmly in her mother or father's arms. Several times I was allowed to hold the baby. I knew then that all the rest of my life there would be a small part of me that would be warmed by the memories of the first moments with Taylor at 10 days old. We thought ahead to times when there would be visits so that we could continue to see her grow.

Some of the dreams of those early sleepless nights were fulfilled in the months and years to come. Charlie and Blyth brought Taylor to Washington and Nantucket. She even came with the whole family for a trip to France when she was six months old. All the early "miracles" happened: Taylor crawled, she walked, she talked, and she was the center of many lives.

Sometime in the autumn of Taylor's first year, we learned that she was to have a first cousin, who would be born the following spring. Charlie's twin brother Tim, and his wife Alison were to have a baby. We were all happy that they would be so close in age, and noted the fact that children of identical twins are really more like half siblings than cousins. Tim and Aliey's baby was supposed to be born in May. Easter was in early April in 1988. Because Easter Sunday is the traditional time to celebrate baptisms in the Episcopal church, the family had gathered in Cambridge for Taylor's christening— but without Tim and Aliey, because the doctor did not want them to travel so close to the time of the imminent birth.

Good Friday evening Charlie and I had a small party for family and friends in the hotel where we were staying. On that night we heard that Thomas Hayden Lord had been born that afternoon, a month early, and that mother and baby were well. He was a big baby, weighing over seven pounds, and no one was concerned about the early arrival. Now we had another reason to rejoice in this occasion.

Once again, as had happened so often in their lives, each of the twins was simultaneously celebrating a significant event—in this case a baptism, and most significantly, a birth. So we went downstairs to dinner full of excitement. There were about fifteen of us at dinner that night. Before we sat down at opposite ends of the table, Charlie and I had a chance to think about a trip to New York to see the new baby. We thought we might leave Sunday after Taylor's christening, in order to have a chance to see the little one in St. Vincent's Hospital before he and Aliey went home to their apartment.

Sometime in the middle of the meal, as we were all celebrating noisily and cheerfully, I saw Blyth leave the table to take a call on her cell outside the dining room. I thought nothing of this until I realized she had been gone about ten minutes. Knowing that Blyth would not stay away that long for any frivolous reason, I went out to see where she was.

When I turned the corner outside the dining room at the hotel I found Blyth. She was slumped down against the wall in the corridor. Her posture alone would have told me that something was wrong, but Blyth was also crying quietly into the phone. I waited until she was finished talking.

I learned that it was Alison who had called to report that the nurses had taken her newborn boy away because they saw that he was having trouble breathing. Perhaps it was only a precaution because of the early delivery, but Alison and Tim were feeling the loss of the precious baby who had already spent a couple of hours in their arms. The next day, right after the christening, which traditionally takes place on Saturday, Charlie and I flew to New York with the hopes of going to the hospital on Easter morning.

On Sunday, we did go downtown to St. Vincent's to visit Alison and Tim and Hayden, as he was to be called. It was an unusual visit. We had to scrub up and don hospital gowns. Tim and Alison were also wrapped in the blue-grey and white pinafore gowns, and only Alison was allowed to hold the baby. She held him close and pulled the striped flannel blanket back so that we could see.

We looked and loved what we saw: a pink scrunched little face with round plump cheeks, lots of black hair, and a definite mouth, identified by both sides of the family as "theirs." By Sunday afternoon, when we were visiting them, Alison had been in the same hospital Barcalounger chair for three days and three nights. They were in a space that was more of a cubicle than a room, but so happy with their son that, when he was allowed to be with them, whatever discomforts they experienced were apparently forgotten, except when the baby was whisked away to the neo-natal unit four floors above.

It was easy to imagine how difficult this was for Alison because even I, the grandmother, longed to be able to hold Hayden as I had Taylor when she was only a little bit older. This time would come soon enough, and the doctors assured us that the baby would be fine. I felt the same sense of confidence that I always had about a new birth. We were only anxious to be closer to this newest member of the family.

2

FIRST YEAR,
FIRST BIRTHDAY

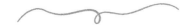

HAYDEN WAS BORN WITH STRAIGHT DARK HAIR AND A TINY red face, usually barely visible in the blankets that swaddled him. His infant colic was so persistent that his father devised a way of being able to eat dinner peacefully, which involved standing at the dinner table holding the baby in a kangaroo pouch with a napkin draped over his small head. Tim would pacify Hayden by doing rhythmic knee bends while eating from a plate held aloft in his left hand. The napkin kept the food from dropping directly on the baby's dark head.

The colic disappeared and so did the dark hair and reddish "old man" look. At nine months, with pink cheeks, golden skin, blue eyes, and white blond fuzz that stood straight up, he looked so like his father and his father's twin that grandfather Charlie and I drew quick breaths of surprise when we had not seen him for a while.

When Hayden was nine months old, we were looking forward to his first visit to Washington. It was exciting to welcome him and his parents to our house. I reveled in all of the crib-arranging and preparations that accompanied these baby visits.

Hayden's girl cousin, Taylor, a year older than he, had come to stay with us at the same age the year before. We put the babies in a room near ours so that we could have early morning time with them, and the parents could get a full night's sleep, often for the first time in months.

When the weekend arrived, we went to the train station to meet the family. They all looked exhausted, especially the baby, who could hardly hold his head up. The noise and confusion of the train had kept Hayden starkly awake for the entire three-and-a-half-hour trip. Hayden, since his birth, had disliked noises and sudden movement. His room was always kept as quiet as possible so that he could sleep. So it is no wonder that both the baby and the parents were exhausted from the trip.

Appropriately for his age, Hayden did not have any words. He did use a number of sounds, which included loving gurgled responses, especially to his parents.

The day after the trip on the train, Hayden still could not hold his head up easily, which his parents attributed to the effects of the long day he had had the day before. The last day with us, after having slept well, his smiles and giggles were more lavish, especially with his parents. We went to bed on that final night of the visit knowing how sad we would be to say goodbye to our beautiful grandson.

When we put this adoring family on the plane to go back to New York that Sunday, I could no longer keep my observations to myself. It only took one glass of wine, while Charlie and I were having dinner at the airport, to loosen my resolve to keep my thoughts to myself. I did not want to worry my husband. This was the first of many meals in the years to come during which waiters, watching us cry, must have wondered what was so very wrong with our lives.

At the same time, we watched happily the pure love that radiated from Hayden's parents. They were so proud of their boy. I calmed myself by realizing that I was, by nature, a worrier. I was the mother who shrieked for help when I saw the slightest blemish on a baby's face, and panicked if a child did not appear to eat enough at even one meal. Hayden's first birthday was coming along in a few months and we vowed to keep our fears to ourselves. Besides, we had hopes that there would be no reason for these worries the next time we saw the baby.

A couple of weeks before his birthday on April 10th, we learned that Hayden's twelve-month pediatric evaluation was scheduled for April 8th. It was hopeless to try to keep my mind on anything else during those days before the doctor's appointment. Charlie arranged for us to visit good friends in Florida the weekend before we were to go to the birthday party. I knew he was trying to distract me and to help us both as we waited for news from Tim and Alison about that check up. While swimming in the Kennedys' pool in Florida, Hayden's golden face was floating with me in the water as I did numerous vigorous laps, trying to tire myself out, so that I might have one good night of sleep.

Back in Washington on Monday morning, knowing that Hayden's appointment with Dr. Goldberg was scheduled for 8:00 a.m., we waited at home for a call. We did not ask Tim and Alison to call us, not wanting to concern them. We knew that no call would be good news.

Some describe these kinds of waiting periods as numbing; I only remember feeling as if electric waves were surging through my body. Charlie and I tried to read sitting next to each other on the couch. I felt sure that Charlie could sense my electric pulses, which I thought would make it impossible to place his thoughts anywhere else—on his book for instance—than that examining office on Amsterdam Avenue.

At 10:30, the phone did ring. Tim was crying as he described what they had heard that morning. The pediatrician told them that Hayden was 6 months delayed. They grasped at the hope the doctor gave them when she said, "With therapy, all the other issues will resolve themselves." We did not ask what the doctor meant by the "other issues," because it was important for all of us to hold onto the shreds of assurance this seemed to provide. Tearfully, yet carefully, Tim and Alison poured out all of the things they remembered from their visit.

Dr. Goldberg said: "He'll need more tests, lots of physical therapy, and we'd advise you not to have another child because this could be genetic."

At the end of our conversation, Tim seemed to be pleading for answers when he said, "How will we feel? What will we do?"

Knowing that we could live up to the answer we gave, we said something like, "No matter what happens, we'll all love him just as much as we do now, and forever and forever."

It was an answer that would prove to have meaning to all of us. In the months ahead, we were guided by Tim, Alison, and Hayden, and Charlie, Blyth, and their children; we discovered that love grew ever more powerful as they cherished and cared for Hayden. Even in the midst of their stunned struggle with this news, Hayden's parents said they would do everything—anything—that would make Hayden well. They would begin by making April 10th a perfect first birthday celebration.

How like Tim and Alison, indeed, to create a party full of smiles and laughter and all the trimmings, only two days after the doctor's dread pronouncements. Almost everyone who was important to Tim, Alison, and Hayden was to be there, with one very important exception: Tim's twin bother, Charlie, who was in Boston. We should have guessed that Charlie would, indeed, arrive to support his brother. The boys had always shared the good and bad moments in each other's lives. One of the "happy sharings" occurred at Charlie's wedding. In this case their father and I witnessed an example of the remarkable telepathic connections that twins share.

Charlie and Blyth had just left their reception and Tim, his father, and I were walking out across a field far away from the tent where music was still playing at high volume. Grandfather Charlie and I were having a conversation with Tim about how it felt to have his brother married. Quite suddenly Tim interrupted and said:

"Charlie is here. Let's go back to the reception."

So, we turned to walk back to the tent in the darkness, Tim very certain of his pronouncement, his father and I very dubious. Charlie was standing in the driveway. He and Blyth had forgotten a necessary accompaniment to any honeymoon—the wallet. Neither we, nor the brothers themselves, realized how vital the confidence and trust of their twinship would be in the coming years, but we could all see the joy that Charlie's presence gave to Tim at Hayden's first birthday party.

At the party, Hayden sat in his high chair, reaching for the candles on his first chocolate cake. He had on a soft cotton suit in a shade of iris blue which just matched his father's and his uncle's eyes. His was a look of baby elegance.

It was a weekday, so Hayden's two-year-old cousin Taylor stayed in Boston where she was in a nursery school. Blyth, Charlie's wife, reluctantly stayed in Boston, too, because she was pregnant and was destined to give birth one month later.

There were a few other children at the party, mostly Central Park friends who had been together during the past year in carriages, then strollers, then crawling, and some walking. We could see that the babies and their mothers and nurses loved Hayden. Bibi, Hayden's nanny, and her charge were often invited to the children's apartments for play dates on rainy days. At these affairs, Hayden sat on the floor when he was feeling strong, though sometimes he flopped over and would have to struggle to get upright again. Meanwhile, the other children reached and crawled and a few eventually walked.

To us and to his friends, he seemed very present in his looking and listening. He appreciated company and people with gentle smiles and small giggles, responding lovingly as he always did when he was held and cuddled. I remember thinking how this first birthday seemed just like any other for a fortunate child of the twenty-first century. Tim and Alison radiated pride and the blue suit got appropriately smudged with the ritual first birthday chocolate. It is impossible to detect any looks of clouded sadness when I scrutinize the many pictures of Hayden's parents and uncle and grandparents that Aliey took at the party.

In the 18th century, first birthdays were honored as significant because so many infants never reached or passed beyond the first year of life. Little did any one of us suspect what Hayden's second year would bring, or how differently we would celebrate his second birthday.

3

A DIAGNOSIS

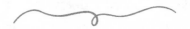

SOMETIME AFTER HAYDEN'S FIRST BIRTHDAY PARTY, CHARLIE and I took a weekend together at an inn in Virginia, where we hoped to indulge in three days of resting and reading. We went on the weekend, having just heard that Hayden had been referred to a neurologist at Mount Sinai Hospital. We had no idea exactly when the appointment was to take place.

On Monday morning, which came sparkling through the rain of the days before, we were getting ready to drive back to Washington. As we were packing and preparing to leave the lovely toile-covered room, we both knew we would be comforted by a visit with Susan Blue, our minister and good friend. Our faith had always been important to us, and had never meant more than in recent years spent in the company of Susan and fellow parishioners. We wanted to say a prayer for Hayden and his parents. We called Susan just before we left, and she asked us to stop at the church on the way home to our apartment.

At the church, Susan took us into the dark sanctuary, where the only light came from afternoon sun glowing through the green-gold Tiffany window, an image of Christ in the Garden of Gethsemane. Susan listened, hugged us, and did not say much. We said a few prayers together. It was, indeed, calming to be in that flickeringly dark space, feeling the peaceful presence that surrounded us. We discovered later that, while we were being soothed in that atmosphere which was both within and around us, Tim and Aliey were with Hayden, who was being examined by the neurologist in a small gray office at Mount Sinai Hospital. This is an office that we would come to know on a cold November day six months later.

We were still unpacking our bags when Alison called to describe the visit to the neurologist. She was speaking in a tense, controlled voice, and I wanted to respond to Aliey's assumed calm by not showing my own quaking feelings. Tim had to go to a dress rehearsal of a play he was in, and Alison was facing this difficult conversation alone. Thinking back on those moments on the phone with Aliey, I realize that it was the first of many times to come when we would find ourselves honoring the courage and strength of our children and their wives. Alison's words, which I tried to record as she spoke, spilled out in an attempt to define exactly what the doctor had told them:

"Hayden has cerebral palsy, diagnosed specifically as spastic dysplasia, affecting mainly his legs. It is a mild case which can range from almost imperceptible to needing crutches. His mind, the doctor feels sure, will not be affected.

It is not genetic. We can have another child someday if we want to. The doctor said to throw away the books on child development. For some reason, he asked us a couple of times about our ethnicity."

When we hung up the phone, after trying—we thought vainly—to murmur words of some comfort, we held each other and sobbed. Then I screamed. Thinking back on these tears and agonies, I realize that I was much more verbally violent in my reactions to those first encounters of sad news than I would be in succeeding years, when the diagnoses multiplied and became ever more devastating. There comes a time when sadness is so deeply lodged that one works from the depths of being to acknowledge the pain, and one lives with a quieter despair.

Shortly after this conversation my reactions were layered with selfish questions and tinged with anger. How unfair! Where is the God that seemed to soothe us in the church only an hour ago? Would Hayden walk, talk, play?

For months, I could not pass a playground without look-ing into the group of mingling children to see if there were any boys with limps or trouble walking playing happily with the other children. Every time I saw a boy with a racquet or a ball I wondered if Tim would be able to play these games with his son. I thought of the beautiful fly rod that Hayden's godfather gave him when he was christened, and hoped, because it was a sport that was done with the arms, that he would be able to go fishing with his father.

I was reading as much as I could find on the subject of cerebral palsy. It was reassuring to read over and over again that the level of affliction with which a child is born does not increase with time. The challenge for the family and the child is to find the best way of compensating with the given condition.

In the midst of all of these doubts and questions I looked forward to summer and to being able to see for myself how Hayden was progressing. In only a couple of months the family would gather at the cottage by the beach. Hayden would be there with his cousins, aunts, and uncles.

Taylor, then two, had a new little sister named Cameron. I longed to see my three grandchildren together and imagined that Taylor would be dodging the waves while Hayden and Cameron were plunked down together on towels in the shade of an umbrella, watching shadows. Our Scottish godchildren were to be there, too, making sure that Taylor remembered to say "bathing costume" instead of "swim suit" and "tea," meaning supper.

As the summer began, the sounds of the older children playing and calling to each other in the yard were just what we had thought summer sounds should be. In the midst of a certain sadness and unease there was humor. Taylor was jealous of her new sister and showed it in distinctive ways, often clinging defiantly to her mother. Once Taylor grumbled:

"I feel mad at Cameron because, well, there's no room for me on Mommy's lap. And, when the baby gets hungry, Mommy feeds her from her boob!"

Taylor was learning to pump herself on the swing, gave many picnic parties from her sandbox and happily named and described the world she was discovering. We were touched by Tim and Aliey's admiration and love for their niece, who was an accomplished two-year-old.

Once, when Taylor was marching, drumming, and humming, and Tim wistfully admired her actions, Charlie's response was: "Hayden will be doing that someday." Tim's answer was "Well, whatever." Maybe he was not so sure.

Tim had already told us that he would take time off in the fall to take Hayden to a special clinic in Philadelphia. We were all watching Hayden, then fifteen months old, and Cameron, who was just four months old. Cameron moved and wriggled and laughed and reached for toys hanging above her bed. She was developing into what her pediatrician would later call "a perfect six-month-old."

Hayden was having a better summer than he'd had the year before, when he was three months old. He did not wake every time a door slammed or a glass was set down on a table near him. He was growing stronger as a result of the exercises that Tim and Alison did with him—exercises they did as often as he could tolerate the work. "Work" it was: pulling himself up on their fingers, grasping and letting go of certain toys, rolling a ball back and forth, and having his limbs manipulated as forcefully as he could bear. All of us tried passing toys back and forth with him, hoping to get him to use both of his hands for play. We were happy when he alternated hands when holding a ball. Hayden, large for his age, continued to grow physically and reminded me of one of the putti, the chubby infant angels painted by Mantegna on the ceiling of the Ducal Palace in Mantua.

Something important happened to me that summer, especially when Hayden was in the room or in my arms. I began to feel that circular, boundless love that makes no judgment. The bitterness and anger gave way to a completely different feeling, something more than acceptance and more than resignation. There was a sense of peace and strength that came from being in Hayden's presence, from holding him and caring for him. This was a feeling completely different from my relationships with the other grandchildren (and my own children as babies). With the others, I was so often watching for growth and change, cataloging new words, actions, and expressions.

There was a mystery about where Hayden would go in this world. Sometime that summer the "mystery" became one of Hayden's gifts. In coming years we learned from Charlie to refer to changes that Cameron and Hayden brought to us as their "gifts."

I was beginning to experience the meaning of unconditional love, which I had always heard of but did not understand. Not being something that one can learn, this state is, indeed, a gift. In retrospect, it was good to have reached this stage at the end of the summer of 1999, because it formed a protection against the stares of strangers and others who did not know him and the occasional hurtful questions and comments that we would encounter in the future. No one who knew Hayden, even for a few minutes, could not help but be captivated by his beauty, his chuckles, and his joy.

4

STILL NO ANSWERS

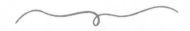

EARLY IN OCTOBER CHARLIE AND I ACCOMPANIED TIM, ALIEY, and Hayden to a scheduled second visit with Dr. K., the pediatric neurologist at Mount Sinai Hospital. Remembering their first visit, how difficult it was to digest the stunning news they received, Tim and Aliey wanted company. They wanted more eyes and ears than their own on this eighteen-month evaluation, the anticipation for which was filled with hope and expectations, and perhaps some undisclosed fears. We all wondered just what the doctor would say, but none of us revealed any anxieties to each other.

Remembering the tranquility of our time together in August, when Hayden was calmed by quiet care, soft wind, and the play of shadows under his favorite tulip tree, I—and I suppose all four of us—found the trip across Central Park in the cab stressful, quite the opposite from our summer experience. Horns were honking and cab doors slamming; motorcycles passed us; and we were even pushed over on the

Park Drive by an ambulance warning. We watched Hayden's peaceful look change as he jerked into a startle in response to each of these intrusions.

As we pulled up to the doors of Mount Sinai, I was thinking of the avowedly modest goals that Aliey and Tim had set for Hayden after the appointment the previous spring. All they wanted, they said, was that by Christmas time, Hayden might be able "do a little crawling and finger-feeding himself". Tim and Aliey, Hayden's therapists, and Hayden—especially Hayden—had worked so hard since April. Still, this little boy, now 19 months old and growing physically in such a beautiful way, was not yet able to accomplish these tasks.

Our visit started in the office, with Dr. K. asking questions in a gentle manner, while watching Hayden, whose plump body was propped on his mother's lap. He was not asking for any reactions from Hayden. He was not directing himself to the baby at all. My memory of the office is that it was grey and lit with harsh fluorescence. Anxiety swept over me as I listened to the doctor's questions. I was overcome by confirmation of the dread that had held me. There were no positive answers to Dr. K.'s questions:

"Does Hayden say anything? Mama? Dada?"

"Does he know his grandparents?"

"Does he hold up his arms to be picked up by his parents?"

Taking our cue from Alison and Tim, not one of us said "No" to any one of these questions. Maybe we murmured something. Maybe we were silent. I could not look at the faces of my son and daughter-in-law. We all knew that the correct answer to each of these questions was, in fact, "No." I tried to look as if I was taking it all in, as if this was a regular check-up. At the same time I prayed that the others were not having the spinning stomach and the weak-kneed shivers that I was experiencing.

After the office visit, the doctor asked if we would move with him into the examining room, where he asked permission to have a colleague assist with Hayden's physical. It was a tiny room, hardly large enough to contain parents and grandparents, the doctor, and a large, gentle, white-coated woman, who we learned was a medical student. She seemed to fill the small space almost up to the ceiling as she loomed over Hayden.

It seemed odd to me at the time that the doctor himself hardly touched Hayden's body. He spoke to him in a very quiet voice, apparently trying to make it easier for the baby to tolerate the young student's examination. She was not manipulating his limbs. Instead, she was looking into his eyes with an oculist's flashlight. Thinking back on these moments, which were difficult for Hayden, it appears that Dr. K. and the intern were possibly looking for "the cherry-red spot" on Hayden's retina, a finding with a significance we would later come to know about.

At the end of this visit, the doctor told us that he would not revise the diagnosis of cerebral palsy that he had given on the first visit until Hayden was three years old. He would see Hayden every six months until then.

We finally found a cab to take us back across the park to 96th Street. Charlie and I sat in the back seat next to Aliey, who was cradling Hayden. We winced to see Hayden's reaction as Tim slid in next to the driver, slamming the taxi door and slumping into his seat. Certainly there must have been other times during the next months when he would show his frustration, but this is the only time I ever witnessed an angry gesture on Tim's part. Aliey was quietly composed. Hayden reflected her calm and his body relaxed against hers. The leaves were falling all around us as we were crossing the park, mirroring that autumn sadness that I was feeling. No one tried to talk or to find the pleasantries that would mask our feelings of disappointment at no new treatments and no answers.

Back at the apartment, Tim sank deeply and silently into the big chair where he always fed Hayden, and where the father and baby son watched baseball games together. On the surface, Alison seemed calm and stoic.

Later, in the kitchen, I tried to say something about my feelings. I wanted to cry, to have us release the tensions and sadness we were carrying within ourselves. I wished that Tim would be able to—would want to—find a sympathetic professional who would help him cope with the turmoil of the unknown they were facing.

We left this visit with no resolutions; and we left feeling that Tim and Alison were struggling with the sensation that things were not progressing as they would if Hayden did have cerebral palsy. Tim and Alison never said anything to us to indicate any worries. The fact was, though, that we had all read and been told that cerebral palsy symptoms that are present at birth do not worsen, but are actually mitigated with exercise and therapy. Later that night, I thought back to our visits in the early seventies to Dr. Davies, our children's pediatrician. He would examine each child thoroughly and gently, then look up at me and pronounce, "A well child."

Later in October, Tim, his father, and I had lunch at a restaurant near Tim's office. By now the leaves were off the trees, but the sun was out and we were eating outside. We had not yet seen Hayden on this visit, so our first questions were about our grandson. Tim's face clouded and his beautiful blue eyes brimmed when he told us that the therapists were being negative about the baby's progress.

At this time in Hayden's life, there were four different people visiting the apartment weekly who, along with Hayden's parents, were filling the charts lined up along the hall with notations and comments about the baby's progress. Tim was getting up early each morning to read to Hayden, to sing to him and play with him—to try to make fun out of the therapy sessions. On the charts (made by Alison), there were check marks to indicate how many times the baby had done his pull-ups (an exercise done by holding the fingers of his father, mother, or therapist, and then pulling himself up, in order to strengthen his back and core), grasped for toys, rolled the ball back and forth to his parents or therapists, and looked up at bubbles being blown over his head. The checks and numerals in the boxes were growing smaller in number.

Charlie thought for a moment after Tim told us about the disappointing reactions from the therapists and then made a calm suggestion about a strategy that Tim and Aliey might use in the next conference about Hayden's progress.

"Maybe it would be helpful, at the next meeting of all of the therapists, to begin by asking the person you find to be the most optimistic of the group to give an evaluation. You could then see where the discussion goes from there. What do you think?"

Tim agreed this would be a good way to analyze the true reactions of these professionals who had been working with Hayden so lovingly and diligently over the past months, and who had been so optimistic about his progress in the beginning.

Later, Alison made a wonderful supper. She is indeed one of those people who manages to do it all, do it well, and make the effort seem graceful. Hayden was pulled up to the table in his stroller. After supper I had the privilege of giving Hayden his night bottle, and was changing him and putting on his footed pajamas. I had not seen many smiles in the past month. At that memorable moment he was cooing and bubbling, smiling and mouthing his loving sounds.

Suddenly, I felt a presence behind me. I put my hand firmly on the baby and turned around abruptly. Tim was there. With tears falling, he said, "Don't let on that I'm here. I don't want him to see me crying."

5

NEWS THAT ONLY COMES TO OTHERS

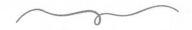

TIM AND ALISON CALLED ALL FOUR OF HAYDEN'S THERAPISTS together. They asked the woman they recognized to be the most optimistic of the group to give her opinion about Hayden's progress. As she expressed concerns about Hayden's condition, the other three therapists entered the conversation. Each of these highly trained people, all of whom cared deeply for the baby they had worked with faithfully for several months, admitted they had given up the hope they had shown for his improvement. The therapists recommended that the baby have an MRI, though they did not say why, nor did Dr. K., when Tim and Aliey asked him to give the order to the hospital.

Several days after the meeting with the therapists, the news came to Tim and Alison, who had spent a grueling hour trying to calm their little boy during the MRI procedure. They called us as soon as they got home.

"Hayden has Tay-Sachs disease. He's going to die. He might live to be five or six."

Once again, overcome with sadness, it was impossible to listen or talk. We could not understand each other's words, much less absorb the meaning of the message. We talked very briefly, if you can call our form of communication "talking." Not wanting to make the children labor over the details, which were still so new and horrifying to all of us, our only recourse seemed to be to try to convey the love that speaks through silence.

Immediately we called Deirdre, the twins' sister. Deirdre was on the computer reading aloud to us, revealing more details about the fatal news we had just heard. We learned that Tay-Sachs is the most common form of a group of autosomal recessive diseases called, collectively, lysosomal storage diseases. Both parents have to be carriers in order for an afflicted child to be born without the necessary gene for the production of an enzyme called hexosaminidase A. Without Hex A, lipids (fatty substances) build up in the brain uncontrollably and cells do not develop normally.

One of the indicators, in the early stages of detection, is the "cherry-red spot" surrounded by a white halo, which is visible when examining the infant's eye. It is this white halo which indicates the pathogenic buildup of lipids, whose presence will eventually destroy surrounding tissue.

Deirdre continued to read. She was unable to bring herself to describe what she was finding. The descriptions of the inevitable blindness, the seizures, the inability to chew or swallow, the assault on the child's respiratory system—it all seemed too overwhelming to describe to us. And these were clinical descriptions, without mention of the kinds of decisions which the appearance of each new symptom would require of the parents.

It was Alison who, several weeks later expressed her reactions to what they had learned: "It's a strange world when you wish desperately that your child had cerebral palsy."

Now that we were aware that Tim and Alison were both carriers of the disease, we also knew that either the boys' father or I was a carrier, and that either Peter or Anne Smith (Alison's parents) must be a carrier. We were confused because we all labored under the delusion that Tay-Sachs was a disease that affected the Ashkenazi Jewish population, and no one in either family was of Jewish descent.

The next day, all four parents made appointments to have "The Test." You do not just walk into the doctor's office to get this test; rather, you must find the nearest acceptable clinic or hospital which is prepared to give the test. In Washington and in New York this is not difficult, as these cities are major research centers for the disease.

In a week or so, I was to find that I was the carrier in our family, and that Anne Smith was the carrier in their family. Amazingly, neither Aliey Lord's mother, Anne Smith, nor I carried the Ashkenazi strain of the disease. Ours, each different from the other, were known as "spontaneous mutations." This is only one of the reasons why our family tragedy was such a rare occurance. The odds of our situation were calculated to be 1,800,000. We would learn later about the complications and errors in testing and diagnosis which affect families in more remote parts of the country.

The weekend after we learned that Hayden had Tay-Sachs, Tim and Alison invited both sets of parents, and Tim's siblings (Charlie and Deirdre), to come for the weekend. We would have dinner Friday night, in what would be the first of many occasions when we learned the power of the support that we could give to each other. The children did not force an agenda; we were simply brought into a circle of concern and understanding, made deeply meaningful by the mystery which surrounded the future of this angelic little boy whom we all loved—our second grandchild, the Smith's only grandchild. The atmosphere was one of challenge and controlled sadness; and there was, to me at least, a sense that we were on the verge of starting an epic communal journey.

I only remember one conversation from the dinner part of the evening: Aliey's father, Peter Smith, gave a toast to Charlie, Hayden's other grandfather. Peter, usually such an affable friend, had been quiet recently, sitting with us but contained in his own thoughts or doing a puzzle. Peter, I know, was mourning as we all were, and was simply present in his own gentle way. Peter's toast thanked his co-grandfather for bringing faith, openness, and ease into this evening of terrible sadness, a beautiful and touching addition to the sad evening.

All day we had been sharing Hayden, taking turns being with him, changing him, and alternately helping with drinks and supper preparation. After the meal Tim and Alison wanted to put the baby to bed by themselves. We left the apartment quietly, hearing Hayden's parents lingering over bedtime stories, prayers, and rituals.

Saturday the gathered family ate lunch while Hayden napped. In the afternoon we all bundled up with warm clothes, tucked Hayden into his blanketed stroller, and went for a walk in Battery Park. We chatted and strolled for fifteen blocks or so and then sat on a bench while Hayden had a bottle. Being alive on such a beautiful day could not help to bury the sadness. I remember discovering that I finally knew what heartache really means; it was as if one side of my chest was actually bigger than the other. I felt a sensation of floating, of otherness. There was physical throbbing and, at the same time, detachment.

While we were on the bench, Tim and Charlie were leaning over the railing, talking as they always have, unconsciously shutting out the rest of the world, identical profiles turned to each other. Later, Charlie repeated some bits of the conversation they had been having:

Tim said, "Sometimes I look at Hayden and I see you and me when we were two years old."

Charlie noted, "I think the cousins, Cameron and Taylor, will be Hayden's best friends."

Finally Tim said, "I'm going to move part of my office to the apartment so that I can do something special with Hayden every day. A week ago I was not sure I could live with this, but now I know I can do it."

Our weekend together ended after Saturday dinner at Tim and Alison's, who were so generous to have brought us all together to help us face this cruel news. Now they needed to have a quiet Sunday with their little boy.

The following Wednesday, the week before Thanksgiving, Charlie and I were scheduled to have our carrier tests. While we were walking son Charlie downtown from 96th Street where he was staying, he did not mention what we discovered later: Blyth was waiting for the results of her Tay-Sachs carrier test, which had been done in Boston earlier in the week. Neither did we speak about the fact that Charlie himself, as an identical twin, was certainly a carrier. As our son turned to go east on 75th Street, I reached up to give him a hug. I remember my words at that moment:

"I hope you never have to see your adult child suffer."

6

A CHRISTENING AND A THANKSGIVING

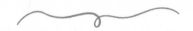

AT ALMOST THE SAME TIME THAT TIM AND ALISON WERE MEET-
ing with Dr. Goldberg in New York to learn more about
Hayden's prognosis, young Charlie and Blyth were in Boston
having a meeting with Dr. Goldstein, receiving the news that
Cameron, now six months old, was also a Tay-Sachs baby. Our
son could hardly speak when he called. The only words I could
understand were, "We're going to lose her. She's going to die."

I remember exactly where I was sitting. I felt like I was
going to slide off of that bedroom chair and not be able to get
up from the floor. Once again Charlie and I were clinging
to each other, feeling helpless, knowing that all we could do
for comfort was to hold onto each other for a few minutes. I
thought, "There is no God; this is the end of our world. How
can we possibly help our children?"

When I think about those moments of blackness the
words "primal scream" come to mind. But I didn't scream.

I was quite silent, only feeling that my body was distended from fighting to contain what it was holding inside.

Two days later, just two weeks after the family gathering in New York, we were to go to Boston for Thanksgiving. Because so many family members were invited for the Thanksgiving weekend, Blyth and Charlie decided to baptize Cameron Patterson Lord on the same weekend. Hurriedly, godparents, siblings, and friends changed Thanksgiving plans in order to be part of the christening ceremony which would take place on Saturday.

When our plane arrived in Boston, we went directly to Charlie and Blyth's house in Cambridge. Taylor, then two and a half, was at school, Cameron napping on the third floor, and Blyth in the living room upstairs. As we climbed the stairs and turned into their living room we found a vivid demonstration of the meaning of "anguish."

When she saw us, Blyth, always delicate and very thin, slid onto the floor, looking like an empty pile of clothing, sobbing and wailing. Pale and wraithlike, it seemed as if she were breathing out her pain. Blyth's usual air of joyful equanimity was gone. She stood up when we came into the room and clung to her husband, then to the two of us. She was not hugging, but leaning into Charlie as if trying to pull strength from her husband's lean frame.

Since Cameron's diagnosis, Charlie and Blyth had been trying to maintain control over such emotions in front of Taylor. So it was important to us that we be part of their despair before we all gained our composure and had to leave to pick up Taylor at nursery school. When we went to bed that night in our B&B, I waited for sleep, torn by the events of the day, feeling the way one does after three days without sleep.

We celebrated Thanksgiving at Blyth's parents' on Friday that year, so that they could include the many family members who were to come for Cameron's christening. On Thursday morning we went to be with Charlie, Blyth, and the children. I ironed the christening dress, which had been worn by generations of family members, including our own three children. I loved the ritual surrounding the christening clothes: opening the box where everything was packed in blue tissue paper; pulling out the dresses and jackets and deciding which ones to use for which baby.

We couldn't use any of the little bonnets for six-month-old Cameron, because the boys and Deirdre were tiny infants at their baptism. In fact, our twins, being premature, were so small that I had made hats out of little handkerchiefs to fit their tiny heads. So I found a special hat for Cameron in a thrift shop. It was an antique white satin cap that had grown creamy with age. Tiny ostrich pin feathers undulated delicately around its crown.

That morning, Blyth and I were sitting on her bed getting all these baby things together with Cameron cuddled between us, having one of our moments of mingled tears and hugs. Suddenly Blyth leaned over and picked up that goose-down hat and plunked it on Cameron's head. Simultaneously we burst into giggles and laughter as we saw this fluffy ill-fitting halo floating precariously above those beautiful blue eyes, momentarily full of astonishment at our antics. This moment of lightness made facing the families for Thanksgiving dinner the next day seem easier than I had imagined.

It was this same morning that I mentioned to Blyth how much Cameron's infant personality reminded me of her own. I said that both had the dispositions of angels. Blyth's response was, "Never again will I read The Littlest Angel. It was my favorite. Now we'll retire it forever."

Blyth's sister Elizabeth wanted to call that November holiday in 1999 "the Non-Thanksgiving." In many ways I found on that Friday Thanksgiving that there was a feeling of hope to be found in the realization that our children were going to give each other, and those who loved them, untold gifts of strength, and even humor, in the months to come. I knew then that we were bound together in a painful, yet fully spiritual, reality.

A remarkable number of the people who were to play significant roles in Cameron's life were gathered that afternoon. In addition to the parents and grandparents, and aunts, uncles, and godparents of the babies, there were two others present who had no idea at the time what significance their skills and spirits would bring to the lives of these babies.

One of these people was the Reverend Eleanor Panasevich, whom Charlie and I had met at a wedding a few weeks before. We experienced almost instantly the feeling of friendship and admiration that often only grows over time. Ellie came over from the Cape on the day of the christening, with only three days notice, to open her little church in Cambridge in order to baptize Cameron. In spite of such short notice, Ellie provided an organist and created an elegant hand-printed program for the ceremony.

Also present that day was Eli Merritt, a Yale friend and classmate of Blyth's and Alison's. Eli, an ordained minister, was just completing a second degree in medicine at Stanford. At this very moment in his career Eli was deciding to focus on "end of life" issues.

Not one of us knew, on this day, what difficult questions the children would have to face in the year to come. Such questions as treatment choices, side effects of drugs, choices of pain medications were all unknown factors and, though no one knew it then, here were the people who could help when even other specialists were at a loss.

Saturday morning, the christening took place at St. Peter's Church in Cambridge. Located near Kenmore Square, St. Peter's is an early-twentieth-century building clad in dark red brick. The building has a colorful interior that's darkly illuminated by some nice stained glass windows. How different from the Georgian, white clapboard, 18th-century church in Harvard Square, with its snowy interior and the Revolutionary War bullet hole in its severely beautiful portals! This is where Taylor had been christened two and a half years before.

Charlie and Blyth did not want to go back to Christ Church because, at the time of Taylor's christening, one of the ministers of Christ Episcopal had objected to the fact that one of Taylor's godfathers was Jewish. St. Peter's and its spiritual leader became an important part of Cameron's life and ours. When our new friend Ellie Panasavich opened the doors of her church for us she became part of the family journey.

For the baptismal service, the families sat in the choir stalls, facing each other, bathed in a pool of light and isolated above the dark and empty pews in the nave. Tim and Alison were cradling a sleepy Hayden. Blyth was holding Cameron, who was playing with her dress and moving her hands and eyes with perfect six-month-old grace. Taylor sat next to Blyth and Cameron with her father beside her. I was next, and then Deirdre and grandfather Charlie.

The hymns were the hardest. When we started to sing "For the Beauty of the Earth," I felt my son shaking. On the other side of me, Deirdre was gripping my arm with both hands. I was quivering inside, but felt strangely in control, as we ended the service with "Ye Watcher and Ye Holy Ones," which had been the processional at our wedding. One month before this day I had felt emptied of whatever faith I had. From this christening hour onward, the empty and lost sensation changed to a feeling of being sustained. Without struggling to find it, I was given the sense that God, who orchestrates neither tragedies nor joys, can be reached within these events as a source of strength.

"Fill her with your life-giving spirit; Send him into the world in witness to your love." The congregation at the baptismal service is always asked to pray for these blessings. The words had new significance when we said them that Saturday morning—meaning we would better understand as we shared the lives of Cameron and Hayden in months to come.

7

COPING

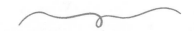

IT IS EASY TO REMEMBER THE SADNESS AND THE TENDER EMO-
tions that went along with the babies' sickness during those
years. It is more difficult to reflect on the angry, violent
responses that each of us revealed. Obviously we were trying
to hide our outbursts from each other, knowing that each
of us had enough to bear. When I think back and read my
journal entries, I find references that help me piece together
threads of these negative reactions.

In my own case, I mention "depression" or "being down"
in my journal even more frequently than I would have imagined. Oddly, Halcy, my therapist, never prescribed medication
for this until late in our discussions. I hid this depression from
myself as well as from others, including Halcy. I certainly tried
not to show the sadness I felt when I was with the children,
but I went to bed crying more often than not. Charlie and I
together, reading favorite passages or saying prayers, would
find ourselves drifting off to sleep on damp pillows. Often

in restaurants we would be struggling to keep back the tears; desserts were often left uneaten. There was one restaurant in particular where the waiters were witness to these "melancholies," and we thought the staff must have sensed that it was either death or divorce that was plaguing us.

Beyond these reactions and tears, my husband Charlie's most obvious symptom of the stress and sadness he felt was that he lost weight, lots of weight. He went to the doctor several times to see if he was physically sick, only to be told that this weight loss was his response to the situation we were facing. He never raised his voice or railed against the injustice we could not help feeling. All of us had differing reactions to these years of sadness, which seems unbelievable as we look back in time. Even Tim and Charlie, identical twins as they were, had quite distinct ways of demonstrating their emotional responses to Hayden's and Cameron's illness.

Tim, as he always had, kept his fears and anguish inside his heart as much as he possibly could. Tim never wanted Hayden to feel his sadness, and was always finding ways to do "happy" things with Hayden: playing games, tickling, watching football or baseball games—always with as much joy as he could communicate to his little boy. When Tim did blow, though, he really let go. He is the one who put his hand through the windshield of his car, venting his rage in private, out of sight of anyone. His gentle response, when he found that his new baby, to be born in October, was a "well" child, was to say, "Our hearts feel lighter now, as we care for Hayden, knowing that we can look forward to and think about the new baby."

Here's one way that Tim, speaking during Cameron's service, responded to the lives of the two babies:

Cameron: You and Hayden were not loud children
in the traditional sense of the word. . . . But in your
untraditional loudness, you taught us how to listen—
not only those of us who were lucky enough to hold you
and read to you and sing to you—but even those who
maybe didn't know you so well. I reckon you taught us
to listen as well, to the joys of the simple things in life
and to how lucky we are for the love that we have. And
for the people in our lives. And for the things we read
that all of a sudden make so much sense to us.

Charlie, Cameron's father, was somewhat of a worrier as a child. He was the one who got stomachaches on Sunday nights before Monday schooldays, and was occasionally known to vent frustration by pounding doors. He, the lawyer, always looked for the facts. He agonized over the research he uncovered when Cameron's illness was first diagnosed: statistics that described the damage that this kind of illness can do to a family. Charlie began his family's journey through Cameron's short life with a determination "to keep and hold the family together in peace." While he continued to be fixed on the small, daily things, such as exactly how much nourishment Cameron was receiving at a given feeding, Charlie sought many of the same sources of support that we all did: his therapist, Taylor's therapist, their beloved minister, reading poetry. But Charlie dug deeper and made life changes for himself by taking on an understanding of Buddhist faith and meditation. Here is something Charlie wrote:

> *On the day that you died, after we played for you "Another Morning," we settled into a complete moment-to-moment existence with you. . . . I existed inside each moment with you, filling each moment with an awareness of being with you and nothing more. . . . Your spirit and mine had fused in a timeless existence that completely embraced the present moment and sent ripples of peace and love down through time, waiting for me in years to come.*
>
> —CHARLES PRIOR LORD, "THE WISDOM AND TEACHINGS OF CAMERON PATTERSON LORD," P. 20

Blyth's strength will be shown vividly when the winter of 2001 is described in a later chapter. In January and February of that year Cameron's illness had taken a major toll. She needed nursing around the clock. Taylor was seeing and remarking upon the changes in Cameron. Eliza Lord was born on February 18th. Grandfather Charlie and I were staying nearby in a B&B so as to be able to help out whenever possible. I never saw Blyth become nervous, irritable, impatient or—least of all—angry. Her almost joyous equanimity did, and still does, provoke a sense of wonder in me. Here is what Blyth said at Cameron's service:

> *Within two days after her devastating diagnosis, I realized Cameron was an angel come to deliver a message*

to me, my family, and our circle. Suddenly the leaves on
the trees were more vibrant in their hue, laughter was
sweeter, tears wetter, traffic irrelevant, people more pre-
cious. In the year and a half since all of us here learned
that Cameron's life was to be short, I know that we
have all—and I mean all of us in this church together—
lived more meaningfully.

It is probably no coincidence that Alison Lord's behavior in response to Hayden's illness was similar in many ways
to Blyth's. It is well known that twins tend to make many
choices that resemble each other—whether they be in work
habits, intellectual interests, or spousal choices. I remember
reading pieces about twins, separated at birth, who insisted
on having a bench around the single tree that each had in
his backyard in houses several states apart from each other.

Alison was a rock of strength. She was affectionate, loving, and patient, always welcoming us, as did Blyth, along with
her own family, for meals or for drop-in time with Hayden.
Alison was, and still is, the most orderly person I know. She
has ideas of how she wants things done and she has control
over her household, her office, and many volunteer activities.
It is no wonder that she was in charge of human resources for
a large advertising company, subsequently started her own
company, and now is an executive at Google.

In many ways, Alison, showing her love for Hayden,
made the most dramatic changes of any of us in her attitude
to life and child rearing. She began life as a mother declaring
herself "intolerant of children without schedules…. I will have

regular sleep times, and there will be toilet training when I decide it is time." Alison and Tim had a particularly difficult task when finding the round-the-clock help they needed for Hayden. Nurses came and went, did not show up, and often had to be fired. Aliey coped and managed with such love for Hayden and in a tempo completely responsive to his changing needs. At his memorial service, Alison thanked Hayden for giving her the patience and the ability "to be a better mother to all of my children." This was a distinctly different response from the plans she had originally formulated for child rearing.

Alison and Tim, Charlie and Blyth, and grandfather Charlie and I would never be able to talk about these times without mentioning one other person who helped us all. Deirdre, Charlie and Tim's younger sister, played a role of such importance that I see her presence in every picture that I have in my mind as I play out the scenes from the Hayden and Cameron years.

During this period, Deirdre lived partly in Boston and partly in New York. Wherever she was physically, she was there spiritually for all of us. She was present with her brothers and sisters-in-law when the new babies were born. She learned as well as the parents and the nurses how to do the complicated feedings and how to administer medication to Cameron and Hayden. It was Deirdre who took on dreaded aspects at the end of the babies' lives: arranging the funeral home, moving the little bodies, going to perform the legal duties of identifying them. Charlie and I thought these would be our responsibilities. Our three children decided they wanted to take this cruel task away from us, and Deirdre insisted that she be responsible. With her usual courage and calm, she made these things happen. We never knew much about her decisions.

In the meantime, Deirdre became the confidante for Taylor, someone to whom Taylor will always turn for help. Eventually Deirdre did volunteer counseling for children whose siblings had died, traveling to Brooklyn one night a week after work to help children in circumstances she had come to understand because of what Hayden and Cameron had taught her. In these capable ways she is her father's daughter.

My comfort during these times came first from Charlie, then from my children and, finally, from reading. There were one or two passages which I read almost every night. Here is one that I cherished:

> *There lies behind everything, and you can believe this or not as you wish, a certain quality which we call grief. It's always there, just under the surface, just behind the façade, sometimes very nearly exposed, so that you can dimly see the shape of it as you can see sometimes through the surface of an ornamental pond on a still day, the dark, gross, inhuman outline of a carp gliding slowly past; when you realize suddenly that the carp were always there below the surface, even while the water sparkled in the sunshine and while you patronized the quaint ducks and the supercilious swans, the carp were down there, unseen. It bides its time, this quality. And if you do catch a glimpse of it, you may pretend not to notice or you may turn suddenly away*

and romp with your children on the grass, laughing for
no reason. The name of this quality is grief.
                                    —JAMES SAUNDERS,
                    "NEXT TIME I'LL SING TO YOU," 1962

At the time when we were reading this, I remember thinking that it would be with me as a constant and ever-present source of meaning: helping, explaining, illustrating what was happening in my life. I still think it is one of the most beautiful evocations of sadness ever written, and it pleases me that Tom Stoppard thinks so, too. But I do not use it, or ones like it, anymore. Perhaps this is because I do not want to be taken back to those times when beautiful sights, mostly familiar ones, were weighted with heartache.

8

TELLING TAYLOR

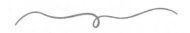

WHEN WE CAME TO CAMBRIDGE FOR CAMERON'S CHRISTEN-ing we had not seen Hayden for three weeks. Hayden, now eighteen months old and the size of a very large two year old, had changed in these intervening weeks. He was calm and seemed to have a distant look of peace and serenity, with which we became familiar as the months progressed. He could no longer hold his head up by himself, and his blue eyes, so like his father's and his uncle Charlie's, were heavy and deeply lidded, a sleepiness caused by the medication used to mitigate the seizures. Around this time, babies born with Tay-Sachs begin to lose their ability to see. Hayden, though, always recognized and responded to people, especially those he knew best. He made his love and personality known with smiles, giggles, and gurgles of recognition, especially when his mother or father read and dramatized a silly story. A picture taken at Cameron's baptism shows grandfather Charlie holding Cameron and me cradling Hayden. We are smiling through our tears. Hayden, looking down, is quiet at this moment.

At the gathering after the service, when someone asked to hold Hayden, Aliey said, "You have to take him from me and hold him as if he were a newborn."

Taylor, at two and a half, talked about Hayden a lot and when she was with him she covered him with kisses. It was apparent that she did notice some of the changes we could see, though she was not alarmed by them. After the service, when we gathered in the undercroft of the church, Taylor looked up at me and said, "Hayden's head is back so far. He has such long, long legs!"

A couple of weeks after the christening, Charlie and Blyth decided to pick a time to tell Taylor about Cameron's illness. Laura Bassili, the counselor who worked with terminally ill children and their families and who was another of "Cameron's gifts," had guided Charlie and Blyth to the strategy of being completely truthful without ever telling Taylor things that she did not ask to hear. Later, Taylor always called Laura "my talking doctor." She called her pediatrician, Dr. Goldstein, "my poking doctor." In quite a matter-of-fact way, she often told people, in her Boston accent (acquired from her well-loved first babysitter), that she had two doctors: "my poking doctah and my talking doctah."

So, sometime after the diagnosis and the service at St. Peter's, Charlie, Blyth, Cameron and Taylor were walking in the Audubon sanctuary. Charlie said, "Taylor, you know how baby Hayden's head falls back a little and how he's big and can't walk?"

"Yes, Dada. He has a disease."

"Taylor, the disease is called Tay-Sachs disease. Cameron has this, too. She and Hayden have had this disease since before they were born. It is not a disease that anybody can catch. It is not anybody's fault and there is nothing that we can do to fix it, but we can keep loving them and taking care of them."

According to her father, Taylor listened but said nothing. After their walk they all went to see a large illuminated tree in Cambridge. Taylor played and chased her mother around the tree, while Charlie sat on a wall nearby holding Cameron and watching Taylor, who had been too young to remember her first Christmas, as she danced joyfully. That night, when Charlie walked into Taylor's room to read her story and put her to bed, she resisted and then began to sob. Charlie, knowing the real reason for the tears, scooped her up into his arms:

"I know, honey, it is scary and sad. You must talk to us any time you have questions about Cameron's disease. Remember, it is nobody's fault."

Then, with Taylor calmer and leaning against him on her bed, Charlie reached across for Curious George. After they read, they snuggled and laughed about the untimely disappearances of The Man with the Yellow Hat and Taylor went off to sleep. The next morning, Taylor came into Charlie and Blyth's room:

"Daddy, I had fun reading Curious George with you last night," words which Charlie took to mean, "Daddy, I felt better after we talked."

A few months later, when Taylor had already asked and been told that Cameron would never walk or talk, she developed a "game," which Charlie and Blyth called "the Tay-Sachs baby game." Taylor would start the game by lying in Charlie or Blyth's lap, saying: "Pretend I am a baby with Tay-Sachs." They were then supposed to say to a pretend big sister, "Big sister, your little sister has Tay-Sachs. Because of the Tay-Sachs, your little sister will never be able to walk or talk. The disease is nobody's fault and none of us will ever get it. Mommy won't get the disease and neither will Daddy. Cameron has had it since before she was born."

Sometimes Taylor would launch into this game when the family was at a party or in a store or at the supermarket. It could happen anywhere. Taylor would collapse and "lose" the use of her legs. As soon as she heard the repeated litany of the reassuring words, she would recover and skip on, or continue with happy conversation.

Throughout the last twenty-two months of Cameron's life, Taylor was the loving older sister; running in after school to give a kiss or to share school projects, or to play simple baby games. When Cameron could no longer play or respond, but lay in her bean-bag chair draped with a soft fleece, Taylor would sing songs to Cameron or put on music for her. She continued to talk to the little one, just as we all did, telling stories and asking if Cameron liked the story, or wondering which music the baby would like to hear. When the seizures began, Taylor was able to do what her parents helped all of us learn to do. Taylor would talk while Cameron fell back into a quiet state: "It will be all right. It will go away. We love you, Cameron."

In the last months, Cameron slept in an elevated queen-sized bed so that a grown up could lie in bed next to her. Over the bed, in front of a pastel quilt mounted on the wall, there was a string of tiny lights and sometimes a candle flickering on the bureau nearby. Cameron never went to sleep alone. We always sensed that there were angels watching Cameron, but just as important to her was Taylor's living presence. The sisters would fall asleep on the vast ocean of that high bed, with blond heads touching, and Taylor's robust pink fist surrounding Cameron's pale hand.

9

CHRISTMAS 1999

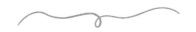

A MONTH AFTER CAMERON'S CHRISTENING CEREMONY AT ST. Peter's Church, the families were gathering for Christmas, which was to take place at our cottage in the village of Siasconset on Nantucket. Every bed would be full and we had borrowed two cribs for the little cousins, Cameron and Hayden. Our Christmases with the complete family were always filled with laughter and many esteemed rituals. The twins, their wives and Deirdre cherished the time together.

Though we did not discuss our forebodings, Charlie and I, and certainly the babies' parents, were fearful that this might be Hayden's last Christmas, and certain that it would be Cameron's last Christmas as a smiling, ostensibly healthy, baby girl. We were all determined to revel in Taylor's pleasures as she enjoyed her first "aware" Christmas. Charlie and I were buoyed by the children's courage, and took heart at the way the boys' twinship and their wives' close friendship helped them all as they moved through these times of sadness and anguished decision making.

On Thursday, December 23rd, while we were waiting for Charlie, Blyth, and their children to arrive, we were trying to get the house ready for the holiday. Grandfather Charlie was putting lights on the tree while I was preparing some traditional favorite foods and stuffing fresh pine branches in all the nooks and crannies of the little cottage. Just as Charlie and Blyth were unpacking their car and Taylor was running up the front steps, Tim called. The boys would often call each other just at the moment when the other boy was arriving for a visit, so I did not find it strange that the phone rang at that moment.

It was not good news that had prompted the call. Hayden was very sick, suffering from another case of pneumonia. His parents knew what pain lay ahead for him, as he had just struggled with his first bout shortly after Thanksgiving. Due to Hayden's traumatic hospital visit in November, Tim and Alison had made the decision to avoid future hospital visits and to keep him at home in his own environment during any future illnesses.

As the Tay-Sachs disease progressed and compromised his central nervous system, Hayden's swallowing reflex and his ability to cough were severely affected. It was miserable for him to feel unfamiliar hands trying to suction and clear his lungs when he was unable to clear the air passages himself. His parents could not bear to see him overwhelmed by the confusion and noise that he encountered in the hospital, where he startled constantly and cried pitifully at these strange and unpleasant surroundings—difficult for any child, but extreme for Tay-Sachs babies.

Tim and Alison had already made some other heart-rending decisions. They vowed that they would never put in a feeding tube, which is sewn into the stomach area so that the baby is fed by pouring liquid nourishment directly into the tube.

Tim said that, in keeping with their overriding desire to keep Hayden comfortable and in his own surroundings, they would not come to Nantucket but would be staying in New York for Christmas. We began to plan a way to make a family Christmas in two places: Nantucket and New York.

There was a way. Within an hour, Charlie was able to call Tim and Alison to say that he had found a pilot who would fly the Nantucket family members to New York. Some of us would celebrate Christmas Eve in 'Sconset, but we would all be together for Christmas Day.

Chartering the plane was the easy part, and we felt fortunate to be able to afford the cost. A place to stay was a different story, however. It was Christmas Eve, after all, and it was almost as difficult to find shelter in twentieth-century New York as it had been in Galilee in the first century. We were too many—a family of eight and two small children—to impose upon any of our friends. Ultimately, Melinda Ely (a former student of grandfather Charlie's when he was headmaster at St. Timothy's School), who managed a small but elegant Midtown hotel, came to our rescue. She was able to provide us rooms, and at a much-reduced rate. It pays to have been a beloved headmaster. Not only did Melinda provide affordable rooms for us, but she even had a Christmas tree lighting our way into the apartment.

On Christmas Eve in Nantucket, we had dinner with pull-pie surprises (tiny wrapped surprises attached to a string, extending from the greens and holly at the center of the table to each person's place), and Buche de Noel for dessert. There were crèches on tables and on the little mantel above the fire: high up this year so as not to be too tempting for Taylor.

After supper, we took a lovely walk in the village, enjoying the views into the few cottages of others who had come back for the holiday. The mullioned windows of the one-story shingled buildings (most of which had been fishing shacks long ago) were lit with candles and we could see the bustle of others preparing their houses for the holiday. The views of these quaint village places are always charming—summer and winter. In fact, the memories of Christmas that year are not so different from other years when we spent the holiday on the island. There are, however, some exceptional and haunting visions, all unique to the year 1999.

Blyth, looking particularly radiant, could not take her eyes away from Cameron who, when not sleeping in her crib, was almost always in her mother's arms. Blyth's expression was melancholy and her eyes sometimes brimmed as she looked wistfully at her daughter. Not wanting to cry myself, I had to force my eyes away from Cameron and her mother. My mind went to the 15th-century madonnas by Ghirlandaio and Lippi, who were often trying to express the emotions of a mother adoring a child who is destined to die. I realized these artists may never have witnessed the sight that confronted us on that Christmas eve. For Taylor's sake, and for our own, we all kept these feeling to ourselves and went on with the traditions we knew and loved.

First we read the passage from St. Luke about the first Christmas, followed by the other selections we had each chosen to read, ones that we had read ever since our own children were small. When the children were small, Charlie and I read to them. Once they got older, Charlie, Tim, and Deirdre each had a favorite passage that they would share. The grand finale is always grandfather Charlie reading "The Night Before Christmas," the same clothbound copy which his grandfather had read to his nine children 95 years before. After the reading of the words "and to all a good night," the children knew they had to run up to bed so that Santa could come. The rush to the covers is accompanied by the ringing of bells that have also served for 95 years.

Early Christmas morning we opened the stocking presents. All of the adults were joyously distracted by Taylor's pleasure, innocence, and lack of acquisitiveness. Before she even saw the tent that she had asked for as a special present, while she was opening her stocking, Taylor said, "I asked Santa for a tent, but I got this elephant!" referring to what appeared to be a special gift: a tiny finger puppet that had been tucked into the top of her stocking.

On Christmas morning at 10:30 we left on the little plane from the quiet airport, its peacefulness a great contrast to the hectic comings and goings of summer traffic. It was a perfect clear and cloudless day. Looking down, I could see deep into the water and recognize the connections between the necklace of islands that flow along the Connecticut shore. Something about the realization of this connectedness moved me to tears as I searched the waters below. It was not unusual for me to experience such intense feelings at nature's revelations during these sad times. The plane trip was another gift that year for all of us, as it brought us to New York in time for the perfect Christmas dinner that Aliey and Tim had prepared.

Just as we arrived at the hotel, however, Tay-Sachs struck another blow—this time to Cameron, who suddenly became very sick with what appeared to be another case of pneumonia. For the next couple of days, Cameron slept in a closet with a humidifier. Her parents were up with her throughout the night, helping her to breathe.

Hayden was better, not coughing so much, though very subdued and sleeping a lot. Hayden had a beautiful rippling giggle, a sound which caused a friend of ours to nickname him "chuckles." In those post-Christmas days it was hard to get one of his sweet smiles, and that musical, gurgling laugh was not often heard.

Remembering back to my first sight of Hayden on December 25th, 1999, I saw what a toll his sickness had taken. He had dark rings under his eyes and he was no longer such a robust two-year-old, but a thinner, quieter, paler little boy. Up until these days in December, to look at him was to see a pink-cheeked plump putto, one who would have fit beautifully into the crowd of little attendants in Mantegna's Camera degli Sposi.

Even when he was not so well I could not take my eyes away from him. His perfect skin, now quite translucent, brilliant blue eyes (Lord eyes, we call them), and lush dark lashes were irresistible. Hayden's smiles, giggles, and determination had always endeared him to everyone who knew him, or even saw him briefly. It was the same with Cameron, although her personality was quite different from Hayden's. She had a gentle, feminine presence, and an unwavering, piercing look that touched us all. Suffering from the same disease, and almost the same age, each baby shone their own light with their different personalities.

As Charlie and I watched the babies that Christmas we wondered how the sight of the ravages of the illness was affecting Taylor, then three. On the plane back to Nantucket on Monday morning, we were reassured when we heard Taylor say to her father, "I love baby Hayden."

Her father asked, "What made you think of baby Hayden just now?"

Taylor replied, "I dreamt of Hayden and his body is funny." Then she repeated the litany that was to console her always: "I don't have Tay-Sachs. Mommy and Daddy, you don't have Tay-Sachs. Only Cameron and baby Hayden have Tay-Sachs. Right?"

Right. Still, a fear was there for us in various forms. Tim and Alison seemed calm in their sadness because they were very clear about the choice they had made for Hayden's care. They were determined to make every moment of their little boy's life as peaceful and beautiful as it could be. Blyth marveled at the serenity of her brother- and sister-in-law. As the year progressed, she and Charlie would create for Cameron what her father called an "arc of life"—a full life, which would have a beginning, a middle, and an end.

Viewed from afar, one could say that this had been a difficult Christmas, which it had been. In reality though, we were given what Cameron's father would come to call one of Cameron and Hayden's gifts. At this point, grandfather Charlie and I, and, I think, all of us, realized we were going to be able to do more than merely exist through the inevitable sadness of what lay ahead. Charlie and I saw before us living examples of an expression which we had never before understood: "unconditional love." We were awed by the strength of all of our children as we saw the work they were doing during these unfathomable events. Having been given these burdens of tragedy, they were creating worlds of peace for themselves and their children.

10

HAYDEN AND CAMERON: THE SAME DISEASE, UNIQUE BABIES

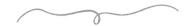

IT WAS A YEAR OF PRIVATE ANGUISH, OF SHARED FAITH, OF torrents of changes, of dying, and of being born. Looking at my journal of these months and reading about the events we experienced, I was compelled to go back repeatedly to check the dates I had recorded. It was hard to believe that all of these happenings were really contained in that one millennial year. It was a year that I had always anticipated as a time of positive change in the same sense that the years 1800 and 1900 had been times of resolution. Certainly this was not to be so in our private lives. Charlie and I took some vacation trips during the year, but our spirits were never far from the sadness that tore at us when we thought of our children and their babies.

As the year progressed, both infants required nursing help around the clock. There came a time when someone needed to sleep next to the little ones, who had been moved to large up-tilted double beds, to help them breathe and release the buildup of fluid in their lungs, and so that a grown-up could lie down beside them. There were sensitive judgments to be made as time went on: about medications for seizures, which developed and intensified during this time, about appropriate nursing care, about creating the most comforting quality of life for these infants as their disease progressed.

Early on that year, I could not rid myself of the fear I experienced when I saw one of the babies having a seizure. When this happened, I always thought of what it would have been like for Tim, Alison, Charlie, and Blyth when they saw those first tremors.

Sometimes we arrived for our visits with the children to find new equipment; sometimes we were present for phone calls and discussions about how to cope with the most recent dilemma. However calmly they were handled, these discussions felt like crises. Sometime during this winter we arrived to find that Hayden had a new carriage, quite different from the familiar stylish and colorful "Perego" type. It was a contraption made of heavy black metal, with rigid padded head and body supports, which could be adjusted to keep the baby's head and body contained, and it was a godsend.

I was aware that on the streets of New York people sometimes stared at us. Once a woman pulled her curious little boy away from the carriage, saying, "No. Come away. There is something wrong with that baby." I felt angry and as if someone had kicked me in the stomach. I only hoped that Tim and Aliey never had to experience such insults.

When we were not with the families, we thought of them constantly, wondering admiringly how they could continue to manage their complex lives full of love, laced with deep sadness.

Prayers, time spent holding the children, the constant attentions of friends, writing in a journal, and reading poetry helped lighten our feelings. We had a folder of thoughts, poems, and meditations that went everywhere with us as we traveled back and forth. Our greatest gift of the year, though, was to come to know the babies as individuals, not as infants who shared an affliction.

During one of our visits to Boston in February, while Charlie and Blyth were reading bedtime stories to Taylor, my privilege was to give Cameron her bottle and put her to sleep or down to nap in the afternoon. I had a special song that came to me then, one which I always sang to her each time we were alone. It was a version of "Lullaby and Goodnight" that included imitations of angels swooping through the air. Cameron loved the dipping loops she saw as the "angels" flew above her.

Cameron was at once gentle, alert, peaceful, and playful. She was a tranquil baby. She moved her fingers, toes, and limbs gracefully, but not rapidly. Her voice was soft and she emitted the perfect contented and evocative coo. Cameron had a stirring ability to fix her searching blue eyes on her mother and father and to similarly engage anyone lucky enough to be holding her. Her father remembers the piercing look that she gave him when he first held her in the hospital. He sensed then, as he held an apparently perfect infant, that she was trying to tell him something. Blyth describes Cameron this way:

> *I am already looking for God in little C. and trusting that he is holding her close. She isn't just mine any-more. I guess she never was—perhaps that explains her near perfection from birth, her adorable noises, her incredible disposition.*
>
> —LETTER TO GPL FROM BLYTH, 1/11/00

In early February, we were with Tim, Alison, and Hayden in New York. Though he had lost the ability to hold up his head, and needed to be cradled like a newborn, Hayden's golden skin glowed and his eyes, which could no longer see clearly, were as brilliant blue as ever. He giggled, chuckled, and made joyous gurgling sounds for his mother and father. His mother could make him burst with laughter when she told stories with her "English" accent.

I can almost relive the feeling of holding Hayden in my arms. Beautiful as he was, he always felt solid, compact, and strong—an odd word to use for a baby who could not move with ease. He was definitely a "boy" baby and also affable, alert, and notably determined.

Sometime during these winter months, I observed some moments which left me with indelible and heart-rending memories. In the living room of Aliey and Tim's apart-ment, Charlie and I were watching Hayden sitting a little unsteadily on the floor very near a large sturdy chest with square "grabbable" handles. While looking at this piece of furniture, Hayden quite purposefully flopped over onto the floor and tried—really strained—to pull himself up on those handles. It was a vain effort; his sturdy body was too heavy and he had to give up the struggle. He released his grip. We watched tearfully; we could sense his determination and his disappointment as his body fell back to its prone position. I do not know if he had done this before, or if he would try it again. We did not ask.

In the spring, Hayden watched baseball games in his father's arms, focusing on Tim's voice as he explained the Mets' strategies. That was one year when Tim never watched a baseball or football game alone.

We cherished these visits, and tried to help as much as possible, though nothing meant as much to the two families as their ability to share their experiences with each other in person. Not only were Charlie and Tim twins who had always had a telepathic connection, but Alison and Blyth were best friends and had been roommates in college and had remained close even before they shared this tragedy.

Once a month, the boys and Blyth and Aliey would spend a night or two together either in New York or Cambridge. Charlie and Blyth could look at Hayden and see something of what lay ahead for Cameron. When they were together, they shared the care of the babies. Sometimes I cannot tell when looking at the photographs of these visits whether it is Cameron's father holding her or her Uncle Tim.

Mostly through e-mail, other Tay-Sachs families passed suggestions on practical methods of care back and forth to each other and to those who were newly afflicted. But I think nothing was as important to our families as what they were able to learn from each other. There were times that winter when we wondered how they would carry on through the intense pain of seeing their children fade and grow weaker. Would there ever again be moments of genuine celebration?

Yes! In February Aliey and Tim told us that Alison was pregnant. This was the first of the few times that we had to wait with very cautious delight to know the outcome of the initial news. In order to be sure that the test of the placental material would give an accurate reading for Tay-Sachs, it was necessary to wait six weeks before doing the test, which involved taking some material from the outside of the placenta.

We went to sleep each night during those waiting weeks with a prayer for a "well baby." During this period, grandfather Charlie and I were invited to go with Tim and Alison to a meeting with Dr. Desnick, a renowned expert on lysosomal storage diseases and Tay-Sachs in particular. The doctor spent two hours with us in his office at Mount Sinai talking about his work and answering our questions. Because our children's cases were of particular interest to the medical community, the doctor himself would do the CVS test, which would reveal whether the baby in utero was afflicted, was a carrier of the disease, or was free of the disease.

Later that week, a few days after he had removed the section from the outside of the placenta (the chorionic villi), Aliey and Tim had a call from Dr. Desnick: "You may buy the bottle of champagne, but don't pop the cork yet!" This was not the last time we were to hear these words. Each time we waited during those intervening days, we tried to suppress our tensions. There was great joy accompanied by equal parts relief—and, of course, excitement—when we heard that this baby was, indeed, healthy. The anticipation during the months ahead was easy to enjoy after the anxiety we felt during those first few weeks and days, and we imagined it must have been the same for our children.

11

TWO BIRTHDAYS

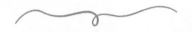

IT WAS THE FIRST OF APRIL, 2000. WE WERE IN NEW YORK for an unusual second birthday. It was a day that represented a spiritual experience and a transformation for the guests, rather than a toddler's tumbling play group. There were no parents laughing, talking, and comparing notes about their children, no tumbling youths crying or falling into each other, and no loud noises or hustle and bustle. It was the most memorable birthday of them all. A friend of Tim and Alison's arranged that we celebrate Hayden's birthday at the Children's Museum of Manhattan, where the hand-colored invitation said we were to be:

In a dreamy forest green
there to find a picnic scene
with a musician and a muse
and any special song you choose.

Hayden had been particularly lethargic because he had not been well for several days before the party. He smiled his little grin, though, and seemed to be lifted by the feeling in the room and especially by the music playing. The rest of us truly were transported to another realm. At that point, the only experience I could compare to Hayden's birthday party was the feeling we all had when Cameron was christened at St. Peter's Church only seven months before.

Cradled in Aliey's arms, then Tim's, Hayden was surrounded by grandparents, god parents, and Bibi (the woman who had helped to take care of him since he was a few days old). A star in the heavens was named for Hayden, complete with a certificate noting its place in the universe.

Afterward, his name was engraved in a painted balloon on the staircase leading to the green, paper tree-filled room where we all sat in a quiet circle, with Hayden at the center. The grown-ups had some sandwiches and cake, while Hayden, who was no longer able to eat solid food, slurped his favorite chocolate pudding from a special bottle. Two of Tim's friends played guitars while we sang—or tried to sing while keeping back tears—the song that someone had composed for Hayden. They called it "Hayden's Song."

Hayden, Hayden, eyes so blue,
Here's a birthday wish for you:
Chocolate pudding all day long,
Lyle Lovett singing songs,
Floating in a bath or pool,
All the things you love to do:

Sitting underneath a tree,
Napping while you feel the breeze.
Mommy singing made-up songs
While Daddy holds you in his arms,
Smelling things that make you smile,
Feeling loved all of the while.
Hayden, Hayden, eyes so blue—
Our love is surrounding you.

Folded on the floor next to each other, so close that we could feel each other's tearful breathing, I feared that everyone present was imagining Hayden's next birthday would be with the angels. Grandfather Charlie and I went back to Washington that evening, filled for days after with the spirit of that hour with Hayden and all who loved him.

Not long afterward, we celebrated another magical birthday, this time for Cameron. We were in Cambridge with her parents, her sister, and both sets of grandparents. Grandfather Charlie and I surprised the children by changing some prior plans so that we could arrive the night before, in time for the party.

These milestone moments held poignant meaning for all who shared in the lives of Cameron and Hayden. Cameron could still sit up in her high chair, alert, smiling, and sensing that the attention was, more than ever, on her. She poked her finger deeply into the chocolate cupcake that Taylor had helped to make. Cameron ate fingers full of her first tastes of chocolate, making a deliciously typical one-year-old's mess in the process. Taylor opened Cameron's presents for her and made a triumphant entry with the balloons. Of course, like most one-year-olds, the single loose balloon was her favorite. Cameron bobbled the string and watched with delight as the yellow balloon responded to her tugs. It was a beautiful day—bittersweet as these celebrations always were—yet filled with many typical moments, which Blyth carefully recorded for the future.

Ironically, these sweet hours with Cameron were taking place at almost exactly the same time that a dreadful experience was unfolding for Hayden and his parents in New York. Hayden had suffered his first grand mal seizure that afternoon. Tim and Aliey did not have the correct medicine at home, so they had no alternative but to take the baby to the hospital.

By the time we talked to them, after the party in Cambridge, Alison, Tim, and Hayden had been in the emergency room at Mount Sinai for four hours. Most of us have suffered the noise and confusion of emergency room care at some point in our lives. It was horrible to imagine what this atmosphere must be like for a baby who startled when a glass was gently placed on a table next to him. The rushing to and fro and the noise and confusion were terrifying for the baby and agonizing for his parents. Tim described the helpless panic he and Alison felt when a mop and pail were slammed down next to the chair where Tim was sitting, holding Hayden in his arms. Naturally, his parents were fearful that these surroundings would cause Hayden to have another seizure.

This traumatic experience helped Tim and Alison and Charlie and Blyth to make a choice that would profoundly affect the remainder of both babies' lives. In subsequent con-versations, both couples decided that they would make it pos-sible to take complete care of the babies at home. Never again would Cameron or Hayden go to a hospital. This was a brave decision; the parents had no idea how to accomplish this goal in a practical or affordable manner. In fact, none of us real-ized what profound meaning this decision and its execution would have to our own children and to the lives of people who would follow this path.

This had been one of the memorable, tumultuous days which we experienced in those years. We knew that Cam-eron's and Hayden's parents sustained many of these days and hours of rapid change and uncertainty. At night, after times like this, when we went back to our hotel, or to our own bed, we wondered and questioned. We would hold each other and ask how these two families could remain together, and strong, through the successions of crises and challenges, while watching the disease take its wasting toll on their beau-tiful babies. Where would we be for Hayden's third birthday and for Cameron's second birthday?

12

SPRING 2000

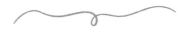

DURING THE SPRING AND SUMMER OF THE YEAR 2000, CHAR-
lie and I spent one weekend every month with Charlie,
Blyth, Taylor, and Cameron, and one with Tim, Alison, and
Hayden. We had taken a break from teaching and volunteer
work so that we could go back and forth relatively easily, and
it was a pleasure to be with the families during these times,
when we could share daily routines—if you can call life with
a Tay-Sachs child "routine."

Easter came in mid-April in 2000 and on that weekend
we were with Charlie, Blyth, and their girls. We went to Easter service at St. Peter's Church, where Cameron had been
christened the previous Thanksgiving, just after her diagnosis.

While all of us were kneeling in a row to receive Communion, I could feel son Charlie's body shaking next to me,
as Reverend Ellie Panasavich blessed Cameron, who was
being held in her father's arms. I tried to whisper something
reassuring, like, "That's all right sweetie. Cry." He said softly,

"I would prefer not to have it be quite so public." There is a small liturgical spoon for removing bits of bread accidentally spilled into the chalice; but there is no such filter for tears that fall there.

These were the months, as we shuttled back and forth, that we wished we lived closer to our children, so that we could be helpful at the spur of the moment. Increasingly, during that year, there were times when crises would arise and we wished we were separated by minutes, rather than by hours.

In early May we were in New York for a few days. I remember giving Hayden his lunch and supper, and Charlie and I were there for his therapy.

Hayden had therapy sessions twice a week—paid for, fortunately, by the generous insurance allotments provided by New York State. The exercises were simple ones: rolling a ball back and forth with the therapists, reaching for objects held out to him, doing stretches, and getting manipulation of his limbs for flexibility.

These workouts started when the doctors believed Hayden had cerebral palsy; in fact, it was the caring young women who worked with Hayden who finally had to admit that the sessions were not helping his "CP," and that the baby needed another consultation with the neurologist. The work that he did while he was thought to have cerebral palsy was good for his muscle tone and his general health. We guessed that this might be the reason why Hayden appeared to be stronger than many Tay-Sachs children we had seen at conferences.

His therapists and Tim and Alison continued to work with him on into the following winter. These sessions were a delicate balance between providing benefits to Hayden and of running the risk of him reaching a state of exhaustion. I will always remember the look of longing in Tim's eyes when he found moments in his day when he could interest Hayden in doing a little therapy work. I could sense his urgent hope as he watched for Hayden's responses to the workouts. Was he getting better at reaching the ball? Could he grasp and hold or tug at a special toy?

Tim could not bear to allow himself or Hayden to give up the struggle. Tim had made an elaborate chart and carefully filled in each day with the number and kinds of exercises the baby had done. That chart was propped up against the wall in the hall of the apartment just outside of Hayden's room. The chart seemed to me to symbolize never giving up. At this point Hayden did not really recognize Charlie and me, though he was full of loving responses and gurgling delight when he saw his parents.

Cameron had her parents and Taylor as her special people. That spring, she radiated whenever she saw any one of them. At that time, Cameron's disease was not as advanced as Hayden's, as we could see when we visited the Lords in Boston, or when they came to us in Nantucket.

In May, Charlie, Blyth, Taylor, and Cameron were in Nantucket with us for ten wonderful days. Cameron was changing slowly from a verbal and expressive baby to a quieter little girl. Though she still ate in her high chair, she spent a lot of time in her reclining seat and in people's arms. This was a memorable visit because it was a particularly happy and easy-going time with Taylor. It was during this week, referring to her pediatrician and her therapist, that she told me that she had a "talking doctor" and a "poking doctor."

One day, Blyth and I, and Taylor, on her tricycle, passed a dead rabbit on the street. Taylor looked at the flat furry animal, quite unfazed, and we walked and rode on. On the way back, Taylor looked again and identified parts of the rabbit. We talked about bunny heaven and I promised I would bury him in a soft place the next day. Blyth began to explain that some bunnies "have short lives, and others have longer lives." Blyth continued on this topic for a minute or two, at which point Blyth and I each received, from this two-and-a-half-year-old, a perfect rendition of what we call the "teenage eye roll."

The next day, Taylor, walking her tricycle, and I, carrying a shovel, took the bunny and put him in a hidden spot in the bushes with some flowers on his body. Later I showed Taylor the spot in the garden under the rose of Sharon bush, where some of our cats and dogs are buried. This all seemed rather interesting and unthreatening to Taylor, but I was surprised that there were not more probings from this very verbal child who, in most cases, was full of comments and questions.

After this visit, we went back to New York for another time with Tim, Alison, and Hayden, and I remember thinking on the plane how good it was that Charlie and Blyth had this lively growing person in their lives while caring for Cameron. While we were in New York for this visit, Charlie and I took Hayden to the Wild West Playground at 96th Street, near their apartment. It was unusually hot that day and we sat under a cooling tree, where Hayden could sense the play of light and hear the splashing of the fountain. He was at his happiest under rustling dappled trees. Years later, a park in the Bronx would be named for Hayden Lord, "tree expert."

We wheeled Hayden up to a bench in his special chair while we chatted with nannies from El Salvador, Honduras, and Colombia—Charlie telling them all about his travels to their countries. A group of sixth grade girls from a local school was having a vigorous water fight and the boys were playing wild tag. Charlie and I took turns cuddling Hayden, whispering to him, and loving the weight of his golden body.

He only had one minor seizure that afternoon, and I found I was indeed able relieve his tensions by using the pressure points that we had learned at the Tay-Sachs conference: steady, firm squeezing on his wrists and a gentle rubbing motion on his chest. Though I had certainly seen Hayden having tremors and then turn rigid several times in the past, I had never actually tried to manage one of these events. Before, seeing the seizures, even minor ones, had always frightened me so that my heart pounded. But this time, I found being able to help was soothing to me as well as to Hayden.

On that perfect June day, Hayden was sleepy, motionless, and silent, even though he was surrounded by laughing, rambunctious children playing noisy summer games. He was still somber and unresponsive when we got back to the apartment. We changed him and gave him some water. What a joy to see what happened when Tim came home from work and picked Hayden up out of his grandfather's lap. Tim swooped the little boy over his head, blue eyes meeting blue

eyes. Hayden gurgled, giggled, and gave Tim a crooked, cooing smile of recognition. Charlie and I turned away from this
evanescent, tender moment, wondering how many more bits
of merriment like this one we would be able to witness. We
would be coming back in a few weeks.

That night, before we left, we planned a dinner out with
Tim and Alison, which was made possible by an institution known as "The Baby-Sitting Club," a group that gave
Tim and Alison a night alone every Thursday. This particular night, Charlie and I were happy to be included. This
generous practice began when eight couples, friends of Tim
and Alison's who were still childless, had arranged to take
turns being with Hayden once a week, caring for him and
putting him to bed, so that Tim and Aliey could have a
"date night" together. These friends had learned, under the
careful tutelage of his parents, how to give Hayden a bottle, give him medications, and get him ready for bed, which
involved putting him into particular sleeping positions that
were comfortable for him. They, too, had learned how to
manage the minor seizures he was having at this time. They
also knew that Tim and Alison were never more than a short
cell-phone call away.

When the four of us were alone, we tried, not always
successfully, to keep each other's spirits up. That night, Tim
and Alison talked about their wonderful therapist, who, quite
by accident, came to be a very important part of their lives.
It happened that an accompanist for a group of Tim's theater
kids, when he heard Hayden's diagnosis, called a good friend
of his, the great Reverend James Forbes, pastor of Riverside

Church. Tim's accompanist friend hoped that Dr. Forbes, known for his wisdom and compassion, would be able to help them deal with their sadness. According to Tim, Reverend Forbes spent a memorable and powerful hour with them, speaking of death and the afterlife, but he explained that he could not do regular counseling sessions.

From among the therapists on the staff of Riverside, Dr. Forbes chose Joan Kavanaugh as the person best able to help Tim and Alison deal with the anguish of Hayden's illness. From that day on they met with Joan, an ordained minister as well as a licensed therapist, every week for a year. Tim and Aliey continued to seek Joan's wise counsel occasionally, after Hayden died. Grandfather Charlie and I met regularly with Joan and her therapist husband before and after Hayden's death. Now, nearly two decades later, I talk by phone with Joan every two weeks. That night at dinner, we had no idea that Riverside, with its graceful replica of the apse of the Chartres Cathedral standing tall on 125th Street, would figure so prominently in our lives during the coming year.

13

TAYLOR AT THREE

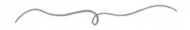

ALONE IN NANTUCKET IN JUNE 2000, I WAS ABLE TO SPEND time with Charlie, Blyth, Taylor, and Cameron. It had been a month since I had last seen the two little girls, both of whom had already arrived at different stages in their lives. Cameron, sweet and gentle as ever, was quieter and less animated. She seemed to smile less often.

Taylor, on the other hand, was more volatile and hilarious than ever. "Miss Jekyll and Miss Hyde" is the way I described her in my journal. I said, "I find her more sparkling every time I see her; it is this spontaneous intelligence that makes her difficult to manage sometimes." In her three-year-old's way, she would balk and refuse any requests from her parents that she did not want to follow. She was more likely to get her own way with her mother, who, by her own admission, tries to avoid controversy whenever possible.

Taylor always insisted that her mother "do cuddle" at night—a lovely tradition which was important in those days when Taylor was so aware of the changes in Cameron. Taylor often cried and did not like to allow her mother to leave the room until after she was sound asleep. In fact, Blyth was kept there so long that she often fell asleep in Taylor's bed. I sometimes became annoyed with Taylor's behavior and was less patient than I might have been.

It was during that week in Nantucket that I saw Blyth display the only moodiness that she had ever shown in my presence. On that occasion, she came into the house with groceries and abruptly dumped the bag on the dining room table. This was hardly a major offense, but it provoked in me a huffy response. At that moment, showing an atypical gesture of aggravation, Blyth quickly raised the baby out of her chair seat and stormed out to the hammock to be alone.

Several days later we learned that there was good reason for Blyth's fatigue and uncharacteristic moodiness. We should also have noted that Blyth refused her usual glass of wine with dinner. Charlie broke the news, and we were able to share, with cautious joy, the prospect of a new baby. We had to contain our urge to celebrate, and be content to feel the anticipation inwardly. We did not dare even talk among ourselves because Blyth had to wait the seemingly interminable ten weeks until she was able to have the CVS test, which would tell her that she was carrying a "well" child. Of course, Taylor could not be told until her parents were sure that the baby would be a healthy one.

It seemed a long wait for Charlie and Blyth but, sometime in July, Taylor learned the news and was as excited and curious as a little girl could be. Taylor, longing for another sibling, could hardly wait to know whether she would have a brother or a sister. One warm, blue day, while grandfather Charlie and I were standing out in the garden admiring the goldfinches swooping back and forth to the feeders, Taylor said, in her Boston accent, "You know how you can tell about the baby? Well, when you change the 'dipah,' if it has a penis it is a boy. If it has a 'gina' it's a girl. Call me whenever you change it if it's a boy." (Charlie and I guessed she was hoping for a baby brother, as she already had a sister.)

In late July, the whole family was together in Nantucket. Those days were full of love and sadness comingled. We watched the young parents cherish and protect their afflicted babies, Cameron and Hayden, and take pleasure in Taylor's antics, while they anticipated the new births. Tim and Alison expected their baby to arrive in September, and knew that the baby would be a girl. As evidenced by Taylor's remarks, Charlie and Blyth wanted to be surprised in early May, when their baby was due to arrive.

We found throughout the summer that it was not only family members who were under the spell of these two lovable little ones. During July and August, when the children were with us, friends and neighbors were in and out of the house. Some people wanted to feel the magic of holding these beautiful children, while others were a little afraid of their delicate states. Hearts melted when we watched Hayden under "his tree," feeling his joy as he absorbed the breezes and the pool of shadows that the giant tulip tree poured around him. Our lovely Amish friend Ruth Anne sat for quite a time, cool in her crisp lawn cap, cape, and blue gingham dress, holding

Cameron, watching her, and looking into her blue eyes. The next day, we received a note from Ruth Anne:

> *Thank you for inviting me to come along with Helen and David to your house. It was a nice party, but what I loved best was to be trusted to hold little Cameron, and to look into her eyes. It was like holding a little piece of heaven.*

Late in the summer we went to help Charlie and Blyth move to their new house in Newton. They needed more space for the new baby and the house was just across the street from Boston College Law School, where Charlie taught at the time. He wanted to be able to come home occasionally during the day to be with Cameron, then fifteen months old.

These months were difficult ones for Taylor. After the closeness of the family summer, she had to leave the only home she had known, and start nursery school for the first time. Taylor was aware of the effect that Cameron had, not only on those who cared for her day to day but on others—strangers like Ruth Anne—who became totally absorbed in the presence of this special baby.

Taylor's anxieties manifested themselves in various ways at this time. Once when Blyth was away for a couple of days in New York to have the CVS test she needed in order to be assured the baby would be free of Tay-Sachs, Taylor woke up at 2:00 a.m. insisting that she see her mother, "NOW, RIGHT NOW! I have to, I have to, I MEAN NOW." Her father's patience and willingness to devote all the time and love required to placate her finally calmed her back to sleep.

Another quieter, but in a way, more dramatic, incident occurred one evening the following week. Blyth's parents, Lyn and Jim Taylor, often generously hosted us while we were in Newton. One evening, we were all gathered in their living room before dinner and before Taylor's bedtime. We were enjoying animated adult conversation. Taylor was on a step at the entrance to the room, looking down at the scene, which included Blyth, who was settled into the corner of a salmon-colored couch with Cameron cradled in her arms. Blyth was looking down into her baby's eyes, and mother and child seemed as one being, surrounded by an invisible mandorla.

Sitting in the chair closest to Taylor, I looked from Blyth and Cameron to my granddaughter up on the step, and saw her face change as she took in the scene. Her features slowly blurred and changed, rearranging themselves into a troubled frown. Suddenly the little three-year-old, who spoke perfect English, was babbling to herself in a language no one could possibly understand.

It occurred to me that perhaps Taylor was showing pangs of jealousy, such as those I sometimes suffered in the presence of my parents and a brother six years younger than I. Or, maybe she was dreading a change she sensed but did not quite understand. There were so many things that a three-year-old might be thinking and feeling. We will never know.

Later, after the children were in bed, Blyth and I went for a walk in the hot starry darkness, where crickets made the only sounds and most of the houses in the neighborhood were dark. I mustered the courage to tell Blyth the reaction I had noticed from Taylor and had the audacity to suggest some strategies for Blyth that would help Taylor through these times.

As a sensitive child myself—six years older than my "perfect" little brother—I was well aware of the physical pain that jealousy can create. It is so like Blyth, with her composed and gentle nature, to listen gracefully to these comments from her outspoken mother-in-law. Daunted as I was at the idea of having this conversation, and shaken by the feeling that I might have hurt Blyth or made her resentful, I was grateful for her unthreatened acceptance of my feelings.

Looking back on Taylor's behaviors during these nursery years, everything we saw should have been expected from a child in her age and circumstances. Here was a little girl growing up in a family willing to share the tragedy of a baby sister who, as she changed and regressed, needed more and more love and care from the very people that Taylor herself loved the most. Her parents were remarkable to watch as they brought her along, giving her the attention, confidence, and support she needed in order to thrive as a student and as a person. In middle school, Taylor was described by one of her teachers, Kathy Coen, as a young woman full of "modesty, warmth, flexibility, and good cheer (who) made our group cohere."

14

HAYDEN HAS A BABY SISTER

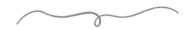

IN OCTOBER, FINDING NURSES FOR HAYDEN BECAME INCREAS-
ingly difficult. Often they did not show up; sometimes when
they did arrive, they could not manage the medical care the
little boy required. Alison and Tim had to suffer the passions
of each crisis that came along. Sometimes it seemed there
were a dozen crises a day.

Tay-Sachs parents from all over the country frequently
communicated by e-mail, sharing struggles and suggesting
solutions for the similar issues they faced. Help from other
parents with comparable problems was especially important
for those who lived away from metropolitan areas, where
families found themselves unable to get appropriate medical
care for this rare disease. Few states offered such generous
financial aid to stricken families as the Lord children were
able to find in Massachusetts and New York.

Here, in one of those e-mails, is how Tim and Aliey (then almost nine months pregnant), described Hayden's needs in September and October of 2000:

Hayden now takes all of his food by bottle—we use a special bottle that has a little vacuum disc that helps bring the food into his mouth when he sucks. It has saved him, and us, a world of worrying. In fact, he gained so much weight when we first started using these bottles ... that Alison actually called the pediatrician to see if he could be eating too much. The best part of this new feeding approach is that we can give Hayden a lot of different taste treats—mango shakes, sweet potato and maple syrup ... Bibi adds yellow peas (a staple of the Guayanese diet) and plenty of savory spices and garlic. Haydoo is a regular "gourmand."

—TIM, SEPT. 2000

I marvel at those who take no medication and wish that could be us, but I am pretty sure that would not be the best for Hayden at this point. Now Hayden's dose involves three different meds five times a day. That's all for me—I ask your prayers that I give birth before falling through the floor to the downstairs neighbor's.

—ALIEY, OCT. 2000

As it turned out, this prayer would soon be answered. The nursing situation on the weekends was the most unpredictable, so Tim and Aliey were reluctant to leave Hayden on a weekend to have the baby, who was taking her time and already several days late. So the parents decided, with the doctor's approval, to induce the baby on October 8th, a Wednesday.

It is no surprise that Anne Warren Lord, whose self-directed independence has since made itself well known, took initiative and arrived on October 5th, unaided by medical intervention and weighing 10 lbs, 7 ounces—more than the combined weight of her father and uncle when they were born 36 years earlier. Tim called us in Washington at 6:00 a.m. that morning and, though our temptation was to rush for a plane immediately, we waited for a reasonable mid-morning departure.

That hour-long plane trip to New York seemed to take twice as long as usual. Unlike our feelings about the births of our own children and our first grandchildren, and even though we knew that Aliey was carrying a "well baby," we were unnecessarily nervous, wanting so badly to have the parents experience an easy birth of a typical baby, who would enter into a household so full of love, yet so busy with Hayden's complex care.

When we arrived in New York, we hurried uptown to Mount Sinai Hospital, carrying our bags with us. We clambered out of the cab, bags and all, and found the maternity ward and a happy and exhausted Alison. Annie, then about eight hours old, was in her mother's arms. This new baby seemed to us to be the plumpest and wisest-looking newborn we had ever met. After a short visit, while Tim stayed at the hospital with Aliey, we went to spend some time with

Hayden at the apartment, where he was in the capable hands of Bibi, who had known him since he was born.

Hayden had a lot of seizures that evening. Sometimes he would stiffen all over his body. At other times he would quiver from head to toe. It was not only agonizing to see what appeared to be painful to Hayden, but these moments were also frightening. My heart pounded each time, with the dread that we might not be able to make him comfortable again. Charlie and I longed to be able to provide a calming presence; we did not want Hayden to sense our tension.

In the end, though my heart was jumping, we did make Hayden comfortable by using all the procedures we had learned at the Tay-Sachs conferences and from Tim and Alison. He knew we loved him, as we had shown all of the times we had held and cared for him, so he helped us by responding to our attempts. We gently squeezed the pressure points on his wrists and massaged his chest, and he slept. When Tim came home, Hayden was peaceful, and gave the lovely murmur of contentment that he saved especially for his parents. That night I asked Charlie to write in my journal. These were his words:

> *I was scared, fearful that we have been so cursed that maybe we would face another blow. Gay and I are both tense and fearful and sensitive, so we have been snapping at each other—I suppose understandable under the circumstances now a healthy Annie has arrived. Thank God; and bless you Hayden for your love.*

That night we shared some bittersweet moments and a few teary ones. Tim, who gave such quantities of teaching and love to Hayden, was reassured to realize that there was room in his heart for both babies.

We stayed in New York for a few days after the birth. Aliey's mother and I had done errands and some cooking to prepare for the newborn's arrival. On the day she was to come home, yet another new nurse had to be found for Hayden. Once again, the expected one had called in sick. The new nurse—named Mary—was calm and capable with Hayden.

The day turned out to be a peaceful one, with none of the confusion that a newborn's arrival can sometimes bring. This tranquility was mostly due to Alison's typically careful organization and planning. In spite of aching muscles after the birth of such a big infant, Alison was her usual graceful, take-charge self.

One of the memorable things we did that day was to prop the two children up right next to each other for a first portrait. Their heads were nearly touching as they lay, each on a large sofa pillow. Annie, the unusually animated newborn, was snuggled into the large quiet body of blond Hayden. Annie's dark eyes were wide open, while Hayden's azure eyes were quite hidden by long lashes drooping with sleep. Sleepy as he was, it was clear to us that he felt the presence of someone, tiny as she was, nestled beside him.

We flew home to Washington knowing that wide-eyed Annie had already brought a new energy and joy to the lives of everyone who lived at 12 West 96th Street. At home in Washington, feeling guilty about being depressed when our children were carrying their burdens so bravely and without complaint, this was what I wrote in my journal:

> *I feel so useless and exhausted, devastated at the idea of facing years more of anguish at watching these babies suffer, and worrying about their parents.... Am just dragging depressed. I do not know what good the visit to Halcy (the psychotherapist) will do. We will see.*

In fact, my meetings with Halcy always helped me move out of the depressed times and on to practical and thoughtful ways of being. Much later I would learn to use meditation techniques to help with these feelings.

There were so many other factors that buoyed our spirits: the thoughtfulness of friends, who would meet us for dinner so willing to listen to these stories as they unfolded; the possibility of looking forward to holidays when the family would be together. We felt a sense of purpose, too, as we discussed the creation of a family foundation intended to grapple with some of the problems our children were facing. So far, the Cameron and Hayden Lord Foundation was only an idea, but it was invigorating to know that there was much work to be done and that everyone would have a part. "At last there is something we can do, something we can help to create," I thought.

Unlike Cameron and Hayden's parents, Charlie and I were fortunate that we could go away for short trips occasionally. Shortly after Annie's birth, we did go away to London to visit old friends. These friends, who were young parents themselves, were full of love and understanding for Charlie and me, and all of the family. One of these dear friends, Julia Ogilvy, would eventually write a book inspired by the lives of the babies.

Throughout this time in our lives, a few words from a sermon, a fragment of a poem, or a small conversation would capture us and would become a momentary inspiration or perhaps enter our prayers. One such moment occurred when we were in London eating lunch at the National Gallery. We realized, as we recognized the distinctive voice rolling out from the table behind us, that we were hearing Sister Wendy, art historian, author, and television personality.

The large, toothsome nun was holding forth in that unmistakable voice, sipping a glass of wine, accompanied by an adoring group of acolytes. She was describing her deep appreciation of St. Paul's letters. This is a fragment of what I overheard:

> *They are enormously touching in their deep sense of loss. . . . I am convinced we will all meet again someday, unless we are absolutely determined to hate God.*

15

SEPTEMBER 2000: NEW YORK AND GREEN-WOOD

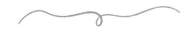

HENRY WARD BEECHER, JEAN-MICHEL BASQUIAT, LEONARD Bernstein, Samuel Morse, Louis Comfort Tiffany, Boss Tweed, and "Bill the Butcher" Poole are all buried in Green-Wood Cemetery in Brooklyn (along with several Civil War veterans in unmarked graves).

Also in this historic and lushly planted ground are members of the Dwight Rockwell family (in a pretty spot inside a slightly crumbled brick mausoleum). Not far from my Rockwell ancestors are the graves of descendants of the Lord family. Old trees tower above their headstones, which are surrounded by a low, ornate iron fence.

Charlie and I hoped that son Charlie, Blyth, Tim, and Aliey would want their babies to be buried in Green-Wood, near forebears from both sides of our family. When we spoke to the children about this, they agreed that the little ones should be buried near each other. They all understood our desire for this.

When they were teenagers, the boys and Deirdre had come up that winding hill to the Lord plot and the Rockwell one, for the burials of their grandfather Lord and uncle Dwight Rockwell. Even Blyth, whose close family members are buried at the family farm in Vermont, agreed that Cameron should be remembered at Green-Wood near her cousin Hayden.

In September, Charlie and I made a trip to Brooklyn to the cemetery, where we hoped to reserve a place for the two babies in the Lord family burial plot, because it is the more beautiful of the two and there seemed to be ample space there for future generations. Under the watchful eye of the official who would guide us to the plot, we were given permission to peruse the old records to find the original purchase agreement signed by Charlie's great-great-uncle Kenneth Lord sometime in the late nineteenth century. Attached to the formal black leather book was a note from Uncle Kenneth, penned in faded brown ink. We were astonished to read the following words:

> *This plot is not to be occupied by any spouses OR children of generations succeeding the children of Charles Edwin Lord.*

We had no idea that this stricture existed. In fact, we were both quite open-mouthed at the news; I found myself pleading with the helpless official for some way to change this edict, which Charlie's great-great-uncle had so unfairly imposed. We had actually contemplated this as a place for many succeeding generations. Our predicament deepened when we were told in no uncertain terms that there were few if any large places available at Green-Wood. We looked at the readily available ones laid out at the edges of the grounds in rows, battlefield-style.

How fortunate we were to find a friend of a friend, who was on the board of Green-Wood, who very kindly paved the way for someone to "find" us three larger plots from which to choose. When we returned to see these a few days later, we got to know the cemetery better, as we wound our way along the roads to inspect the three available locations.

The next time, Tim would come with us, as Charlie and Blyth needed to stay in Boston and had given him their proxy to make the choice, immersed as they were in a household which included a toddler and the exhausting and exacting care of little Cameron. We saw one place we liked, which was on a grassy hill, with a tree and a distant view of the city. It reminded us of Hayden's tulip tree in Nantucket.

We had our minds set on the tree-shaded spot, even though it came with a large underground concrete mausoleum, which had to be removed at great expense. Of course, they did not tell us about this subterranean problem until we were sold on the beauty of the location. We would wait for a final decision until we could show Tim all three of the locations later in the month.

We were back in New York during the last week of September, when we planned to take Tim to Green-Wood.

Early in that week, we spent time sitting near Hayden and reading to him, and just being a part of the gentle care that surrounded him. Hayden was having more frequent seizures by now and was sleeping on his back, propped up by pillows. Breathing was more difficult for him. His delicate rib cage was flared open like a flower trying to catch the sun.

One night that week, we sat on either side of the big bed with our grandson between us quietly watching his thinner, yet still golden, body and the movements of his breathing. With tears welling up in our eyes, we both hoped that Tim and Aliey would not catch us in this reverie, knowing that they must have many of their own moments just like this. Later that night we went to bed thinking of our visit to Green-Wood with Tim, which would take place the next day.

It was a perfect blue and gold autumn day, which began with a visit to one of the schools in the Bronx where Tim was teaching a class to sixth, seventh, and eighth graders. He perfectly captured his hopes for the students when he made reference to this quote from Martha Graham:

> *There is a vitality, a life force, an energy, a quickening*
> *that is translated through you into action and because*
> *there is only one of you in all of time, this expression*
> *is unique.*

At lunch, after the school visit, we sat outside at a restaurant near the Museum of Natural History, with its grand trees and flower borders. Now, years later, when I pass that café, I remember the texture of our conversation. Charlie and

I did not try to describe the places we had seen at Green-Wood. I remember finding it hard to eat while thinking of the piece of ground that would hold a child who should have his whole life stretching before him. We talked about this sadly as we also mulled over the importance to each of us of finding a hallowed space for Hayden and Cameron, and for future generations.

After lunch, Tim drove us to Brooklyn, leaving behind the sunny café to wind through traffic, under bridges, and past some of the darkest parts of the city, eventually driving along the street lined with the usual monument sellers and florists displaying Technicolor plastic bouquets. Finally, the road opened to face the imposing, yet curiously welcoming, red-stone Victorian entrance gate, and we could see through the dark entrance to the light-filled trees and sky beyond.

We were met by a man from Green-Wood's staff who was to drive us along the roads that wind in and around the grave sites. Many times I had been driven on these complex routes, which contribute to the mystery and beauty of the place. I remembered well the distant views of New York and Battery Park across the sparkling river. Only this time did I notice the Statue of Liberty holding court in New York Harbor. Not surprisingly, like most older ladies, her beauty is best appreciated from afar. After climbing from the drive to the prow of a hill, we came to the spot where the cherry tree was bowing over the open green space. Just as we hoped, this was Tim's choice, too.

In the car on the way back to the city, we talked tearfully about our reactions to this visit. Tim remarked how strange it felt to know exactly where he would be buried. It made us realize that our son, at 38, was still too young to be contemplating his own mortality with the same degree of acceptance as his nearly 70-year-old parents. My perspective was that I was happy to know where I would "be."

All three of us agreed that we were glad that Hayden would have his tree. Now we would think of this tree as being a part of Hayden's world, as is the tulip tree in Nantucket. A couple of years later, a bench would be given in memory of Hayden near his most convenient entrance to Central Park. His godfather and other friends placed a plaque on the bench which reads, "Hayden Lord—tree expert."

16

NOVEMBER 2000: CHANGES; ANOTHER THANKSGIVING

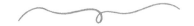

WE RETURNED FROM A TRIP TO EUROPE IN EARLY NOVEMBER to a country suffering a post-election crisis. Florida's hanging chads were flying in the news, symbols of many weaknesses that appeared to be shredding the fabric of the democracy we admired. The crises in our children's lives were also beginning to deepen.

When we called Tim and Alison from the cab on the way home, they told us that Hayden had lost eight to ten pounds in the last month, and that he was sleeping much more now. Meanwhile, Annie was already smiling. When we got home, new pictures of the two were waiting for us: the blond two-and-a-half-year-old, his blue eyes hooded with sleepiness, and the dark, wide-eyed one-and-a-half-month-old, already trying to lean forward to her brother as he sank back into the cushions. We learned that Hayden's somnolent, heavy-lidded eyes were a result of the anti-seizure medication which he took more frequently now.

A little later, when we got to the house, we talked to Charlie and Blyth and learned that Cameron had already taken her first seizure medication. This is how her father described those first seizure moments:

> *Cameron's last physically communicative act was to reach up and stroke my cheek. She did it during her first seizure. As it went on and on, she looked deep into my eyes with that look of peace and wisdom. She rolled over as the seizure continued and reached out and caressed my face. I stopped crying and just held her. Finally, one morning in the late fall of 2000, as I danced with her in my arms she reached up slowly and stroked my cheek. Time stopped. I knew in my heart she would never be able to do it again.*

A few days later, on a cold Saturday night in November, I was at home alone, nursing a cold and reading by the fire when the phone rang. It was Tim calling, saying that Hayden had pneumonia and had stopped breathing for minutes that afternoon. Our young son, the man who had so often astounded us by the composure he was able to muster in front of us, sounded so frightened. Never had I felt a more powerful wish to be able, at that very instant, to hold my grown child in my arms.

Tim and I talked several times that night before Charlie came home from the theatre. Among other things, I learned that one of the nurses had harshly confronted Tim and Alison, saying: "He cannot get his medication. He's coughing and needs a tube." In every one of these situations, the parents had to describe the decision they had made, trying once more to make the nurses understand their need to reject the suffering that comes with tubes and medical procedures and hospitals. Every one of these explanations was accompanied by guilt and, more powerfully, by the realization that, as parents, they are never really ready to give up. In a poem he wrote eight years later, Tim talks to Annie about this period of his life:

> *Holding my breath,*
> *I take you into my arms and roll backwards onto the moss.*
>
> *If I could choose, I would stay, I would come at*
> *   Christmas time and*
> *stoke the big stone fireplace and light the tree for no one*
> *   but the*
> *lonely boat far out on the lake to see.*
>
> *We would come with you and it wouldn't be lonely.*
>
> *We wouldn't think about choice and the irony that*
> *   choice hurts so*
> *much you can't believe that someone would believe they*
> *   have the*
> *right to tell you not to do it.*
>
> —TIM LORD, "CHOICE," 2008

Sometime during that week, after these talks with our children, we realized we had been living in a state of denial for several months, believing the impossible: that we would have Cameron and Hayden for a long time and that their parents could have them, though sick, for a long time. Only a little over a month before, I had written fearfully about "bearing years" of sadness. On the plane to Boston, Charlie and I talked about the time we had left with these beloved children and realized that we needed to revise our sense of time; we needed to be able to cherish fragments of time. The expression "living in the moment" had explicit meaning now.

When we arrived at Charlie and Blyth's house in Newton, we found them in the midst of a crisis. Now it was Cameron who was having an apnea seizure just as we were arriving at the airport. Cameron had stopped breathing for a measureable number of seconds. It being Sunday, Charlie and Blyth could not reach their doctor immediately.

Fortunately, Charlie and Blyth had prepared themselves for emergencies by having special medications in the house. They were on the phone with Tim and Alison, who were exhorting them not to take Cameron to the hospital. Instead, Hayden's parents, speaking from experience, were leading Charlie and Blyth through the procedure for administering anti-seizure medication by suppository, and suggesting that Cameron have a dose of Klonopin, which was also on hand. Though the tranquilizers made Cameron limp and sleepy, she was free of seizures.

Charlie and Blyth were relieved that Taylor, who had spent the previous night out with Aunt Deirdre, and was sleeping late, had not seen the seizure nor the terrified reaction of her parents. We realized that this was the second time that the weekend before Thanksgiving had been ill-fated for our family. The year before, we had been together after hearing of Cameron's diagnosis; we could not help remembering the love we found as we rallied and braced ourselves and gained from sitting tightly together at Cameron's christening.

These days in Newton were also peaceful as we waited to fly together to New York for Thanksgiving. We drove Taylor to her nursery school in Cambridge in the mornings, then came back and spent time holding Cameron in our arms.

The calm of these days was only broken when we arrived at the airport to fly to New York: Both father Charlie and grandfather Charlie were subjected to a random bag check while we were waiting to board the shuttle. As a way, undoubtedly, of releasing the pent-up tension related to seeing the changes Cameron was enduring, and of traveling with a three-and-three-quarter year old child and a very sensitive one-and-a-half-year-old, both men gave forth outbursts of indignation, and more. I referred to this afterward as "the bag-throwing incident." This all passed quickly and we boarded the plane, where I had the chance to hold a quiet Cameron in my arms.

Our time in New York that Thanksgiving can be characterized as a roller-coaster ride of conflicting emotions and memories. There are some beautiful recollections of those days and nights, and some gut-tearing ones. Hayden lay in his big bed (queen-sized so that an adult could lie next to him) with oxygen tubes in his nose. He had pneumonia and sometimes coughed for hours at a time.

In my memories of Cameron, who was rendered limp and pale by medication, she was always held by her beautiful mother in such a way that they seemed to form one body, with Blyth's eyes focused dreamily on her daughter. The sight was reminiscent of a painting of the Madonna and Child with the infant splayed across the Madonna's lap as a prefiguration of the crucifixion.

I remember that, during one long cuddle with Hayden, when I was reading The Old Turtle to him, I suddenly feared I might be squeezing his delicate body too hard. At this very same moment I could hear people in the next room helping Cameron pass through a seizure.

For joyous memories, there are visions of all of us and Miko, Deirdre's kind and wonderful boyfriend at the time, gathered around the Thanksgiving table. Annie was there, either in the musical swing or being passed around from eager arms to eager arms. She was a highly animated six-week-old, set in particular contrast to Cameron and Hayden, rendered so silent by their affliction.

We grandparents enjoyed a long-planned morning with Taylor at Radio City, where she leaned forward in her seat, keeping time to the Nutcracker dances and delighting in the Rockettes' antics. On Thanksgiving Day itself, Taylor was equally delighted to be able to peer out of the window of the apartment that Charlie and Blyth had been lent by cousins, watching the parade with Snoopy and Clifford the Big Red Dog bobbing by, almost at eye level. The men watched football together, something they had delighted in for years. While all of these things were going on—football, seizures, nurses' ministrations, kitchen noises, and other conversations intermingled—I did overhear one conversation between Blyth and Taylor:

"Mommy, Cameron and Hayden look alike."

"How do they look alike?

"Well, they have blue eyes and little noses and blond hair."

"Anything else that you can think of that makes them look alike?"

"Well, they both have eyes that do this," Taylor rolled back her eyes to demonstrate, "and they can't hold up their heads so well."

"Can you think of why?

Taylor, whispering very quietly: "It's the Tay-Sachs."

"That's right. But you don't have Tay-Sachs and baby Annie doesn't. Neither does Le Petit." ("Le Petit" is how Blyth referred to the baby that would be Eliza, who was due in early 2001.)

"I know. There are some good things and some bad things."

While listening to this conversation, I was looking across the room at our two grown sons, dressed up in their Thanksgiving garb and wearing the family tartan vests. They looked so handsome. Typically, they were completely absorbed in each other's company. At these times it was hard for anyone else to "get in" to their consciousness. Their focus was impenetrable and stunning as each boy held his own very sick child in his arms.

Only grandfather Charlie and I realized how much

these babies, sick as they were, looked like their fathers at the same age. This was, indeed, one of "the bad things": wondering if Charlie and Tim would ever again be in the same room at the same time holding their beloved babies in their arms.

17

HAYDEN: BEFORE CHRISTMAS, 2000

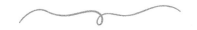

IN OUR FAMILY, WHEN WE GET TOGETHER FOR A HOLIDAY, IT is not unusual to see the three siblings, Charlie, Tim, and Deirdre, slide away from the gathering to spend time together—away from the group. Sometimes they take a walk, or go fishing for the afternoon. Sometimes they have a meal out together.

We did not know, until a couple of weeks after Thanksgiving, that Tim and Charlie had spent some hours together on one of these walks, during which they saw a red-tailed hawk flying over their heads. Mentioning this almost in passing, they nonetheless described feeling a certain mystery in this presence hovering above. Most importantly though, it was on this walk that Charlie absorbed the decisions Tim and Alison had made for Hayden's future care.

Although Tim and Alison had finally found two loving and capable nurses, everyone who was involved with Hayden

was in anguish when they saw the little boy gripped in coughing episodes and battling to breathe, as he lived through
another episode of pneumonia. On this afternoon walk, Tim
described their plan for Hayden's coming months. They had
made the resolution that Hayden would never be allowed to
suffer another bout of pneumonia. Here is how Alison, in
early December, described their thoughts, in a letter to other
parents of Tay-Sachs children:

> Hayden came down with pneumonia the week before
> Thanksgiving. It was the worst two weeks of our life
> together—He would cough for two hours at a stretch—
> We would do chest PT, suction, use the nebulizer . . .
> try warm baths, massage, inverting him, sitting him
> upright, you name it. We had many conversations
> with our doctor asking about ways to make him more
> comfortable, but—because we had not had an explicit
> conversation with her about palliative versus curative
> measures, we talked around the issue, but not about it.
> "No" was the answer when we asked for cough medicine
> with codeine (the cough is "productive"), "No" was the
> answer when we asked for morphine (we are not "at
> that stage yet").

> He has rallied incredibly over the last few days eating
> (not eating as much as before, but that's ok), giving
> us a few "agoos" and breathing comfortably. . . . We
> believe that each crisis we have faced over the course of
> Hayden's Tay-Sachs has prepared us for the next. In

*this case, Tim and I are now on the same page about
what we will and will not do to "treat" Hayden in the
future, and all of the nurses that are helping us to care
for Hayden are on the same page as well (some thought
we could cure Hayden . . .). It is all about comfort. There
is no such thing as a productive cough. We all have to
respect Hayden's wishes and answer to his cues—And
no one knows better than we do what he wants and
needs. We are meeting with our pediatrician to have
a dialogue about caring for Hayden from now on, so
that we are not trying to make decisions in the midst
of a crisis and so that we are ready for the next one. We
are happy to have another chapter with Hayden—and
at peace with the fact that we are ready to let go when
Hayden is ready. . . . Love to you all.*

—DECEMBER 5, 2000

In October, Alison had said, in another letter she wrote
to the Tay-Sachs families:

*When I am in his presence I just see my child that I love
so, so much. It is hard seeing him suffer.... [We need] to
give him the dignity and choice he deserves to decide
when it is time.*

—OCTOBER 4, 2000

And so, after Thanksgiving 2000, we went back to
Washington, understanding their decisions. During these
times our friends would call, often to suggest nights of quiet

dinners. They knew what was going on with us. Part of what I remember of those months when we were at home was the strength we gained from the presence of people who knew exactly what to say and what not to say. Obviously, asking questions and listening comprise a large part of the "what to say" approach. Examples of comments from the "what not to say" group included didactic words from advice givers and such remarks as, "Wouldn't it be just as well for you and the parents of that poor child if he just died soon?" During these weeks we went on with our lives: theatre and book clubs, walks and dinners together (where we invariably got teary over our martinis, a libation which in those days was still one of our indulgences).

One thing we did not do that December was to bring out the Christmas decorations and pleasurably place all the traditional objects in their appointed places. We didn't, as I recall, talk about not performing these rituals. We just did not even bring the boxes down from the attic in the first week of December, as had always been our custom. Our hearts would beat faster every time the phone rang, knowing what our children might have to tell us.

On Thursday, December 14th, the call came. Arriving home from lunch, we found a message from Tim saying that Hayden was suffering another bout of pneumonia. He was receiving baby doses of morphine, as needed, and a valium suppository; and the palliative care person from Mount Sinai had visited. Tim said he and Aliey were at peace, as they carried out the resolve they had carefully deliberated over the past months. They would stay in touch with us every day. They wanted both sets of parents to come when the end was near.

Deep valleys of sadness marked the succeeding days. Tears welled up, especially when I was alone—in the car, or in the shower. At other times, I found it was possible to be thinking of Hayden, and the terrible void he would leave for his parents, and at the same time talk about him in a matter-of-fact, normal tone.

There was an added comfort in our lives during that week. Deirdre, who lived and worked in Boston, happened to be in DC on business. We learned for the first time that our strong and courageous daughter, in order to help her brothers, had volunteered to assume some of the most frightening tasks surrounding the anticipated deaths: to identify bodies at the funeral home, sign cremation papers, and more—tasks which remain a grim mystery to me.

In their wisdom and kindness, our children decided that it was not for grandparents to manage the details surrounding the deaths of grandchildren. Deirdre told us about this while the three of us pondered questions we were having as we waited for more news from Tim. For a moment I felt wronged by this decision, thinking that these duties should have been our burden. This feeling passed when I thought about the times that our sons and daughters-in-law, in the midst of their own struggles, had spoken or written to us about our sadness. To this day, we do not know the details of the responsibilities that Deirdre carried out in the last days of the babies' lives. Even from afar, Deirdre was an important presence for us, and now she had decided to stay on in Washington with us, knowing we would soon have word about Hayden.

On December 15th, a Friday, I was at a friend's house sitting around the dining table reading poetry, with ten friends who met once a month. When the phone rang, I knew it was Charlie. When our hostess answered, and confirmed my fear, I asked her to say that I would be right home. I did not even speak to Charlie. Feeling sick and shaky, I was mute as I gathered my things up from the table and hurried out.

At home, Deirdre, Charlie, and I heard from Tim and Alison that they knew that Hayden was "ready to die." He had taken no food since Wednesday and had hardly accepted any water since Thursday. We were ready to go to New York. Would we leave immediately, go Saturday, or would we wait until Sunday?

We flew up the next morning. We were not afraid of what we would find, as we knew that Tim and Alison were not just resigned; they were calm and at peace as they gave their little boy every ounce of love and care that anyone could have. We had a moment to visit with the new nurses and learned from them that they felt they gained their strength from something invisible that emanated from their quiet little patient.

When we went into his room, we found Hayden propped on his pillows wearing a crown, given to him by his dignified, fatherly African nurse, Benga, to celebrate an honorary chiefdom. The name Benga bestowed on Hayden was Chief Malyegun. A Yoruban word, Malyegun means "an individual that brightens the world by his act."

18

PEACEFUL SORROW: "HEAVEN LIES ABOUT US IN OUR INFANCY"

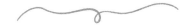

WE COULD SEE THE CHANGES IN HAYDEN'S BODY WHEN WE arrived. His eyes were still blue, but paler, not as azure as they had always been. He was thinner, so thin that every rib stood out and his rib cage flared open, flower-like, to welcome every breath he could catch. His color changed each day as he grew paler; and his skin was pellucid as it stretched over his little bones. His right hand, especially, was pale and blue-white, while his left hand still held the color of life.

All day in the small apartment, various family members were in and out. During the day, Bibi was almost always there with three-month-old Annie, and Benga, Hayden's African nurse, to help with his complex care. Medical procedures occurred on a regular basis.

Despite these comings and goings, a sense of peace, love, and order filled the rooms. For that week, their house had become a sanctuary and the place where we all wanted to be. All of Hayden's things were kept exactly as they had always been. Even the large chart, drawn out in Tim's hand, which he had made to record the progress of Hayden's various therapies, still leaned against the wall outside of Hayden's room.

The two in-law families established a routine so that there would never be too many people in the apartment at the same time. The Lord and Smith families took turns staying with Tim and Aliey to cook meals and to eat with them. When we were there, we had time to be with Hayden, lying down quietly next to him on his big bed, hearing his breathing, and reading to him.

Everyone who came chose bits from The Hobbit. I read some poems and Old Turtle. Grandfather Charlie read Goodnight Moon. Usually Hayden was asleep and very still, with his eyes closed or partially open and looking somewhere else. Charlie and I sometimes told him that it was all right and he could go when he needed to. We were sure he could feel our presence. We spoke softly, even though the little boy had lost most of his hearing. Once, though, when Tim came in and spoke to him in a normal voice, Hayden turned his head to his father. Hayden's bedroom was always very warm; suddenly the room felt warmer.

When Charlie and I did go out for a meal, it felt strange to be with people, or in a place where others did not know our "real life"—the one that was going on at 12 West 96th. I found myself feeling isolated; not wanting to be with anyone who was not part of the circle of emotions that contained Hayden at its center. Here is how Tim's brother Charlie described these days and nights in the writings he did the year after the babies died:

Hayden's night nurses were not so reliable. Hayden's wonderful day nurse, Benga, came in the morning, but from 8pm until 8am we cared for him ourselves—Deirdre and I, Alison's sister and her partner Denise, and Tim and Alison. . . . We manifest the inner spirit by stopping and listening and being still: "Be Still and Know that I am God". Yet through the night I was so nervous. I worried about Hayden being uncomfortable and I worried about whether I could help him.

The next night I gave him morphine (by suppository) at 3:00 a.m. as he began to cough. He was still uncomfortable as the night wore on—and several times I had to suction him and clear his throat for him. Finally at 3:45 a.m. it occurred to me that maybe the morphine had not worked. I opened his diaper and there it was. I re-administered it and he was fine in a few minutes. I lay down with him as I realized that I had so much to say to him. I talked with him about what he meant to me . . . I thanked him for the love, peace, and lessons we had shared since I started spending more time with him—especially the deep understanding I could communicate with him and with Cameron just by being with them and meditating. As I drifted off to sleep next to

him, I began to speak with him about fear. He told me
there was nothing to be afraid of, that there were three
possibilities: 1) That he would continue to be comfort-
able, 2) that he would need my help to be comfortable,
which would give me a chance to show him how much I
loved him and to participate in a sacrament—a sacred
moment of caring, touching God by caring, or 3) the end
of his life would come and he would be at peace. This
was his great gift to me, for I was never afraid about
the last days of Cameron's life or about watching her
die. I was able to tell Blyth about that night and she
was never afraid either about the last days.

—CHARLES PRIOR LORD, "THE WISDOM AND
TEACHINGS OF CAMERON PATTERSON LORD,"

DECEMBER 2001

Blyth, who found it excruciatingly difficult to leave
Cameron in those days, especially with Charlie gone for the
week, also came to be with her nephew. She and Taylor drove
to New York from Boston for a short time. It meant so much
to have them there, even for a brief visit. Taylor had spoken
to Deirdre that morning on the phone, when she had said: "I
spit up twice this morning, but I'm still coming to New York
to say goodbye to baby Hayden."

They only stayed for a few hours, but Taylor never for-
got this goodbye. The next day at 4:00, a letter and a picture
arrived from Taylor, who dictated the words to her babysitter.
The letter was addressed to her father: "This picture shows
you driving to say goodbye to baby Hayden because he is

going to die. You are holding a balloon . . . Sorry I have to go to lunch and a movie with Mommy now."

Memories of this sweet visit stayed with us that week. As the days passed, things happened that gave us the sense that special powers were at work in our lives. Son Charlie described one of these happenings:

> *Every day we walked in the park and looked for*
> *the hawk. On Thursday afternoon, it was clear that*
> *Hayden would die that day. We were at peace and*
> *we had all told him what we wanted him to know....*
> *Deirdre, Miko, and I left the apartment to give people*
> *some space. Miko asked how far we were from Straw-*
> *berry Fields.... As we passed Strawberry Fields we*
> *started to head uptown, but I said, "Let's walk to that*
> *pond." As we came to the pond, I felt a deep calm and*
> *the world slowed down. I looked up and there was the*
> *pale hawk, sitting quietly in the tree above me.*
> —CHARLES PRIOR LORD, "THE WISDOM AND
> TEACHING OF CAMERON PATTERSON LORD,"
> DECEMBER 2001

Sunday of that week, we went for a walk in the park after two dark, rain-drenched days. While we walked around the reservoir, the sun burst through and a triple rainbow appeared. People were turning and looking and exclaiming all around us. I heard one man say, in a distinctly New York accent, "I've never seen a rainbow like that here!" Another morning I was looking for Wordsworth's "Ode: Intimations of Immortality from Recollections of Early Childhood," trying to find this beloved passage:

> *But trailing clouds of glory do we come*
> *From God who is our home*
> *Heaven lies about us in our infancy!"*
>
> —WILLIAM WORDSWORTH,
> "INTIMATIONS OF IMMORTALITY," 1803-1806

A letter arrived that very afternoon from Charlie's close first cousin, Philip. The piece of paper that slipped out of the soft blue envelope contained the very ode that I had been thinking of that morning. We were not searching for these signs. They simply happened.

In fact, most of these days were spent in a quiet routine that had evolved, until Thursday, which was different because people realized Hayden's breathing had changed and his color had taken on a shining pallor. He had deep, dark circles under his eyes. His parents knew it would be his last day, and we left the apartment at midnight with that full and aching feeling that comes with sorrow, leaving son Charlie, Deirdre, and Miko settling into the armchairs and the couch in the living room.

Before we left, we watched Tim and Alison carry Hayden into their room to sleep between them in their bed. Annie was already asleep in her crib on Aliey's side of the bed. There were candles in Hayden's room all that day, and they moved with him into his parents' room at the end of the corridor. His long, thin little body glowed, translucent in the candlelight.

Tim called at 5:00 a.m. to say that Hayden had died at 3:30. Annie woke them with her crying, which was unusual for her at that hour. When they looked over at Hayden between them on the bed, they saw him take two deep breaths, and give a great sigh. With the sigh, they saw him go and knew that he had died peacefully, as they had wished. Tim said that, while they waited for the doctor to come, they all got up and made waffles. "But," he said to us, "we're hungry again, so Dad, will you come and make your scrambled eggs?"

Arriving at the apartment about 6:30 that morning, Friday, December 22nd, first we held each other in tearful, wordless love, then we held Annie for a moment, and put her back in her crib. After this, we heard something about what had happened during that long night. At 4:00 a.m., when Deirdre could not get an answer at the funeral home that had been recommended to them, she called Frank E. Campbell—the only other funeral home name they could remember. Then Tim and Alison took Hayden back to his room and bathed him and rubbed him, as they always did before he went to sleep. Sometime later, Frank E. Campbell answered the call by sending two somber men, dressed all in black, to perform the necessary duties.

Charlie made his special scrambled eggs. We took our plates and scattered ourselves around the living room to eat. I remember it being very quiet for a moment in the room, almost hushed. Suddenly, to our surprise and wonder, Tim and brother Charlie jumped up from where they had been sitting on the floor next to each other, went into the hallway and out the door of the apartment.

We heard timid knocks on the door, which then opened to show the two lugubrious undertakers, as played by the brothers. They came one behind the other at first, then side-by-side, bowing and bowing, removing their pork-pie black fedoras, saying over and over again, "Sorry for your troubles. Sorry for your troubles. Sorry for your troubles." The laughter started in the living room, turned the corner, rolled past Hayden's room and down the corridor towards Annie, peacefully sleeping throughout.

19

FAREWELL AT GREEN-WOOD, CHRISTMAS 2000

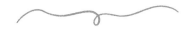

THE DAY AFTER HAYDEN DIED, DEIRDRE, MIKO, CHARLIE, AND I went home to Washington. When we arrived, the house at 45th Street seemed empty. Even though Hayden had only been there once, it seemed as if he should have been there, too.

I had no desire to celebrate Christmas. Later Friday afternoon, after we had unpacked, Charlie began making frequent trips back and forth to the attic to bring down boxes of ornaments and decorations. All the traditional old favorites began to appear: a yellowed plastic musical church from the 1930s that sat under the tree, the angel for the top of the tree, the tattered ornaments glued together by various children—all emerged from their boxes.

When Charlie handed me my old favorite, the wax infant Christ in brocade swaddling clothes, even I realized that we needed to create a special time for Hayden, and for ourselves. Was there a tree in the library already? Probably not. Did we get one the next day? No one who was there can seem to remember. It was so like my husband to rise above his own feelings to bring joy to the rest of us.

Reluctantly, we made the house beautiful and cooked for Christmas Eve and Christmas Day, and as we did we were comforted. We went to church on Christmas Eve and the candles blurred and swam before my eyes, especially during the moments when the lights dimmed during the singing of "Silent Night," the final hymn. Miko and Deirdre helped us with everything we did.

This was the week that so many beautiful and helpful letters came pouring in from our friends and relatives. The letters continued for weeks and months afterwards, and they have been kept as a source of solace since then, in a black leather box on a table in our library. I felt then that the letters themselves could be the subject of a book. We didn't have time to appreciate them at first because we were soon back in New York for Hayden's burial.

Only a week after Hayden died, we were staying in the Lucerne Hotel on 79th Street and Amsterdam Avenue. We never stayed there again. The Lucerne's ornate, incongruous, redstone façade still makes me jump when we pass the building on the way up or downtown; it stands as a memorial to some of our saddest times.

The night before the funeral, we were at Aliey and Tim's

apartment, where we exchanged a few presents. Before dinner, Tim took us into Hayden's room. We saw the bright blue wooden box they had made, which would hold Hayden's ashes, his African crown, and some of his toys, including his favorite blue dog which always lay cuddled next to him. When Tim handed me Blue Dog, I lifted it to my face; it still held Hayden's particular soft smell.

We found Aliey pale, exhausted, and quieter than I had ever seen her. Little Annie was a magnificent distraction for her mother and for all of us, with her smiles and easy disposition. She seemed a definite little being, reminding me of her mother. I thought about that family of three as we went about the few preparations we planned for the burial.

We found a florist so that we could bring pots of colorful primroses to brighten the stark cold surroundings, and four little evergreens, which would eventually be planted in the corners of the green space where Hayden would be buried.

We needed to have a car for the five or six members of the Lord family who would be making the trip to Brooklyn. I had imagined an ample sedan, but the hotel insisted that we would need a limousine, asking, "Would it be all right if we provided a white limo?" The answer from me was a definite and unpleasant-sounding "NO." Somehow, the idea of a white stretch limousine became an excuse for me to become intransigent and outraged. I actually had a crying fit at the thought.

As we went about these small tasks, I had the recurrent feeling of wanting to withdraw to the apartment where we had been together during the week before, the world that included the living Hayden on his big bed, lying next to his blue dog. I wondered whether the burial at Green-Wood would lead us to a level of acceptance of our goodbye to Hayden. I dreaded that this would not happen.

The night before the service was long and dream-filled and so cold that we could not even open the window. The freezing night air seemed to come in through the walls. In the morning, we talked to Blyth, who would leave Cameron for a few hours to fly to New York for the burial and then return home immediately after the service at Green-Wood, taking a taxi to and from the cemetery and the airport.

When we arrived in the lobby in the morning, bringing our yellow, purple, and red potted primroses and the four small trees, we were met by the concierge. He pointed out the windows of the revolving doors to show us our waiting car. What we saw was the whitest stretch limousine one could ever imagine. It seemed to me to extend the full length of a New York city block. I behaved abominably and was still fuming when we piled ourselves into the despised vehicle. Unfortunately, the inside of the car was also memorably offensive: The leather seats were redolent of stale smoke; the cut crystal and bar set clinked, shone, and jangled annoyingly all the way to Brooklyn.

The big limousine pulled up to the ornate gates of Green-Wood at precisely the moment that Blyth's cab arrived from the airport. When I stepped out of the car and looked across at Blyth, I was astonished to see that she was laughing uncontrollably. I blurted out: "Why are you laughing?" Hardly able to contain herself, Blyth explained that the vision of her discreetly dressed mother- and father-in-law emerging relatively gracefully from the glaring white vehicle was so incongruous as to set her into hysterics.

Tim, Alison, and Annie were already waiting in their Jeep in which they had carried the blue box. Led by a car driven by someone on the cemetery staff, we fell into line behind two other cars containing Aliey's family and wound our way up the hills to the grave site. The cold was more biting and the wind stronger as we neared our place, situated as it is at one of the high points of the cemetery.

At the site, the cars parked down on the road below the burial spot. We left little Annie, wrapped in a creamy white wool shawl, in the arms of the chauffeur of the long gleaming limo–its one advantage was its warmth. From the roadway we climbed the steep little hill to the flat place where the bare, twisted branches of the cherry tree leaned down toward the gaping dark hole in the left corner of the green space. The blue box was so far down, so far away.

The Lord and Smith families formed a semicircle around the hole, huddling next to each other against the cold. I was between Miko and grandfather Charlie. We all needed each other then, in so many ways. Joan Kavanaugh, Tim and Aliey's minister and therapist, led some prayers. Afterwards, each of us said something to Hayden, then placed our words or poems down into the hole on top of the blue box. Most of us do not remember what we said, but my journal of that night says that I quoted some of Wordsworth's words, including from "Ode on Intimations of Immortality from Recollections of Early Childhood":

Our birth is but a sleep and a forgetting:
The Soul that rises with us, our life's Star,
Hath had elsewhere its setting,
And cometh from afar;
Not in entire forgetfulness,
And not in utter nakedness,
But trailing clouds of glory do we come
From God who is our home:
Heaven lies about us in our infancy.

After the poem, I prayed that "some of that nebulous grace would remain with us forever."

Grandfather Charlie chose part of the John Donne prayer that we had often read together in the previous years:

Bring us at our last into the house and gate of heaven,
where there shall be no darkness or dazzling . . .
but one equal eternity, in the habitation of thy majesty
and of thy glory, world without end.

When this fell down onto the blue box I could see that it was written on a postcard picture of trees blowing in the wind—such a fitting image for Hayden.

Tim was the last to speak. When he stretched down into that hole, his body told us how much he wanted to be near his boy. He was perched on the edge and leaning way over and down, so that his blond head disappeared into the darkness. Tim returned Hayden's Blue Dog, gave him a star, his horse, and his blanket, and finally a Mets ticket, which fluttered below to rest on the box. Most of us picked our way down the hill to the cars. Tim and Alison stayed by themselves for one last moment with Hayden.

The rest of the afternoon is a blur, but we did go back to the apartment on 96th Street, probably for lunch. As Tim walked into the apartment, he looked through the entry into the hall outside of Hayden's room and said, "Hayden's chart is gone. Who moved Hayden's chart?"

20

JANUARY 2001

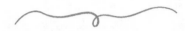

WE SPENT NEW YEAR'S EVE THAT YEAR AT THE HOMESTEAD Resort in Hot Springs, Virginia, with Deirdre and Miko. It was impossible to celebrate in a traditional sense, but we were happy to be together and to be taken care of in the comfortable, traditional Virginia ways. Along with the copious amounts of food and drink that were proffered, there were always opportunities to walk up into the fragrant piney hills for exercise and renewal of our spirits.

There was, for me anyway, a terrible feeling of not having said goodbye to Hayden, compounded by the sense of sadness and concern about the uncertain months that Cameron would face in her life on this earth. How would Charlie and Blyth manage Cameron's illness with the love and attention that they provided so beautifully, care for a new baby, and be able to support Taylor, now almost four?

It was comforting to talk to Tim, who called on New Year's Eve to say that the day before he had gone to a Knicks game with friends, and Aliey went to New Jersey to be with a close friend. When they saw each other late that night they realized, as Tim put it, "Haydoo would not want us to mope." They knew that the deep sadness would come, and felt no need to mourn in dramatic or forced ways. Alison was very private about her feelings. It was hard for her to grieve openly, but Charlie and I knew they were grounded in their love for each other.

So we escaped for a few days into long chilly walks, reading, and occasional games of tennis. When the time came to go back to Washington, we thought we were ready for a few days at home before going to New York for the memorial service for Hayden.

In fact, coming home that January was difficult for both of us. We had been comforted by Deirdre's presence for several weeks and missed her and our conversations with her as we all remembered Hayden. I had recurrent dreams about the little boy, mostly happy dreams of him lying in a tree-filled place with light dappling over him. When I told Tim about my dreams, he told me about the vision he saw in his dream the night that Hayden died: the sweet blond boy was laughing his inimitable giggle in an "eye" surrounded by a cloud.

Tim and Alison spent that week after New Year's planning a memorial service for Hayden with their minister and therapist, Joan. They were calling the service "A Thanksgiving" and their courage made us strong as we faced another trip to New York.

The morning we were to fly to New York, I heard on NPR the voice of Eleanor Roosevelt saying, "Do the thing you cannot do. . . . Every time we live through fear, we can do better next time." Somehow these words said to me, the one who always used to cry when speaking about someone I loved, or reading a poem, or giving a toast, that the spirit of calm and faith that prevailed in our lives in those days would give us strength for the future—and to say graceful words in Hayden's memory. And so it was.

Riverside Church, built in 1930 by John D. Rockefeller, and modeled after the choir of Chartres Cathedral, is an inspiring design. As noted in a 2009 New York Times article, it was also inspiring in other ways: "It stood for many years at the most heavily trafficked juncture of religious faith and social activism in the United States." This is where Tim and Alison had been helped and counseled by Dr. Kavanaugh during the previous years, and where they had gone to Sunday services, usually holding Hayden in their arms. Large as the congregation was, this place of diversity and great beauty felt comfortable for them, as it did for us when we visited.

The original plan for Hayden's memorial service was that it would be held in a smaller chapel with capacity for 300 people. It soon became clear, as people called from everywhere to ask about the time and place of the service, that there would be more than 300 people attending. Tim and Alison heard from doctors, nurses, people from their workplace, performers, friends from all over, and members from the large network that makes up the Tay-Sachs community. Therefore, the memorial would be held in Riverside's large and beautiful main sanctuary, where we gathered on January 12, 2001.

Having gotten to the church early, Charlie and I and the other members of the family sat in the front pew, listening to the organ. As we sat, we could sense that a crowd of people was arriving behind us. Turning once or twice, we could see that the huge space of the nave was filling with people, a few of whom we recognized as good friends and relatives we did not often see. Blyth and Charlie were nearby, Blyth holding a pale and somnolent Cameron. Bibi held Annie, with Tim and Alison on either side, and Aliey's parents were near their daughter.

The tone of the hour was set at the very first moment of the service by a rousing gospel prelude: a rendition of St. Christopher's hymn. The women singing had been coached by an artist who worked in Tim and Jason's Dreamyard program, and they had asked especially to sing at the service. They filled the great space with rolling and swaying sound and movement.

Joan Kavanaugh led the service, which included readings from the Bible: the story of David's son who died ("I shall go to him, but he will not return to me") and Paul's letter to the Romans ("neither death, nor life, nor angels, nor rulers…nor anything else in all creation will be able to separate us from the love of God. . ."). To end the service, Joan read Psalm 139:

> *Lord you have searched and known me. You know*
> *when I sit down and when I rise up. . . . How mighty*
> *to me are your thoughts—they are more than sand. I*
> *come to the end—I am still with you.*

Then family and friends spoke. Grandmother Anne Smith shared a favorite of hers and Hayden's: E. E. Cummings' "Maggie and Milly and Molly and May." Jason Duchin, a godfather, read Pablo Neruda's "I Will Come Back." Brothers and sisters and grandparents spoke about their memories of Hayden's gifts. Alison thanked Hayden for making her "a better mother to all of her children."

There was a video that showed pieces of Hayden's life, including memorable moments of Hayden's giggle as he listened to his mother reading in a silly English-accented voice. Finally, everyone tried to sing Hayden's birthday song. By the end of the song, most people, even the many who had not been present at Hayden's second birthday, were barely able to mouth those final words: "Hayden, Hayden, eyes so blue, our love is surrounding you."

The program announced that a benediction would end the service. It was a musical prayer given by Joan Kavanaugh's husband, a dear friend. Joan led her husband, who is blind, halfway down the aisle, where he sang a Navajo chant, a cappella. His beautiful voice filled the church. It was over.

Driving away from the church that afternoon, we had gone about two blocks south on Riverside Drive when we saw—flying directly in front of us, above the middle of the road—a red-tailed hawk. He stayed with us until we turned east to go to Winston and Bette Lord's apartment for the reception. These sightings always lightened everyone's spirits; we had not seen the hawk since the week that Hayden died. And we did not see him again that winter, not even the following Sunday, when Annie was christened at River-side at 10:00 in the morning.

At the christening, the family sat in the exact same seats where we had been several days before for Hayden. Some of the most beautiful words in this service are the ones sur-rounding the Thanksgiving over the Water:

> *We thank you, Almighty God, for the gift of water.*
> *Over it the Holy Spirit moved in the beginning of creation.*
> *Through it you led the children of Israel out of their bondage*
> *in Egypt into the land of promise. In it your Son Jesus*
> *received the baptism of John and was anointed by the*
> *Holy Spirit....*

When I heard this familiar prayer again, it brought back the words by Neruda, read for Hayden less than two days before:

> *Some time...*
> *when I am not alive,*
> *look here, look for me here*
> *between the stones and the ocean...*
> *here I shall be again the movement*
> *of the water, of*
> *its wild heart,*
> *here I shall be both lost and found—*
> *here I shall be perhaps both stone and silence.*
> —PABLO NERUDA, "I WILL COME BACK"

Reading these pieces together makes it seem no wonder that our friend Julia Ogilvy calls December 21st and May 9th (the dates of the deaths of the babies) Hayden's and Cameron's "Rebirth Days."

21

FEBRUARY 2001:
TAYLOR, CAMERON,
A NEW BABY-AND BELLS!

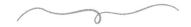

ONE DAY DURING THAT ICY, WINTER FEBRUARY, GRANDFATHER
Charlie and I found what we thought would be the perfect
place for a two-week stay near Charlie, Blyth, Taylor, and
Cameron, while they awaited the birth of the new baby. The
little house, on a street behind the town hall, had a cozy attic
bedroom, a small kitchen and living room with places to read,
and skylights that allowed the winter sun to pour in. What
we did not know when we chose the place was that the bells
of the town clock sounded every hour throughout the night.

There was a lot going on in Blyth and Charlie's house
during those weeks: preparations for the new arrival, four-
year-old Taylor's anxious anticipation, the complex care of
Cameron, and the comings and goings of nurses to help with
Cameron's daily routine.

Maybe it's because Newton Corners is the smallest and most far-flung of the several Newtons; for whatever reason, the village appeared to want to proclaim its existence loudly and firmly with those hourly clangings of its town clock. Insomniac that I am, nights during that period were sleepless ones. We were busy, though, and felt alive because of the swirling energies of care and expectation that were connecting the occupants of the house at 21 Rochester Road.

To us, the daily demands and routines of the household seemed overwhelming; to Charlie and Blyth, this life was what they later termed "the new normal." Cameron's care included meticulously slow and deliberate feeding techniques, sensitive use of seizure medications, massages, and as much time as possible just being near her—singing to her, stroking her pale blond hair, or lying next to her delicate body in her double bed.

Taylor, at four, adored Cameron in a remarkable way. She fully appreciated Cameron's special limitations and was loving and solicitous of Cameron's needs. Cameron's great uncle had made her a unique play station: a small piece of furniture that supported Cameron in an upright position and allowed her to keep objects within her reach so that she could easily touch and enjoy them. After school, Taylor would spend hours in a sunny corner helping Cameron with her activities.

During these weeks, before the baby was to arrive, Taylor wanted more of her mother than it was possible for Blyth to give. Blyth insisted that, after the baby's birth, she was going to come home after only two days in the hospital. When Taylor heard this, she began to accompany one of her occasional meltdowns with loud protestations of "I cannot wait two days!" Once, the nurses reported hearing Taylor muttering, "I hate this house, and there are too many people here."

During these waiting days, Charlie and Blyth seemed to move through the time with focus and ample love to give to each other and to Taylor and Cameron. Who was I, then, to be anxious? In fact, I longed for some of their calm. While the bells rung the hours all through the night in the B&B, my dreaded anxieties kept time with the clapper in the tower.

It is no surprise to learn that the calm that we observed in Blyth was summoned from deep within her, and masked some of her real feelings. On the 17th of February, the day before the baby was to be induced, Blyth admitted she was "scared that something will be wrong." She said, "I'm afraid to look at the baby." I can feel again, eight years later, the turn in my stomach that I felt when Blyth spoke those words.

Recently, Blyth discussed the baby's birth with me. At first, Blyth said she "wasn't worried at all. Every day was a leap of faith." Feeling that I had to be honest with her about what I had recorded in my journal, I quoted these words to Blyth. She responded, "There was continuous grieving and anger about Cameron that co-existed with the anticipation for the new baby, and my love and admiration for Taylor. I always felt so betrayed by the fact that I was nursing Cameron, who had just been pronounced 'a perfect six-month-old,' when I learned that she would die."

I think these fears vanished when the baby was born, on Sunday, February 18th, 2001. Elizabeth Dwight Lord arrived at 3:00 in the afternoon, a healthy little girl—so healthy, in fact, that she was put on display that afternoon for first-time parents, as the "bath demonstration baby."

Meanwhile, at 21 Rochester Road, Deirdre and Miko (who had spent the night with Cameron and Taylor) and Charlie and I were trying to manage Cameron's care at a time when she seemed very uncomfortable and edgy. We sensed that she was experiencing pain and suddenly realized, to our dismay, that there was no seizure medication in the house. And it was Sunday! Somehow, Deirdre reached the pharmacy and Dr. Goldstein, who—in his inimitably reassuring way—managed to get the needed prescription. By the time Blyth came home with Eliza—yes, after only two days—Cameron was again in the routine of care that made her peaceful.

There was a glow that radiated from her room at the top of the stairs, where there was a string of lights and candles, and delicate mobiles turning and dancing. Cameron, in the midst of the big double bed, with her golden hair catching the soft lights and her pale skin shining, did not need to say words to demand attention. These were cold days outside, with snow piling upon snow. But we were warm inside; Cameron's presence was the central fire in our lives, while Taylor provided the essential spirit.

We imagined that the days after the new baby came home might be daunting—maybe even chaotic. In fact, those first weeks with Eliza, Cameron, and Taylor were peaceful because Charlie and Blyth made them so. The gentle and reliable nurses were there, as was Tanya, the capable au pair, who was a familiar presence. Before we turned down her light, Cameron's father would sit in the big chair next to her bed reading On the Day You Were Born, while Cameron lay in his lap and I held her delicate hand.

We took turns sleeping with Cameron, lying next to her in her big double bed. The first night that I took a turn, I wondered if I would sleep, or ever relax. I wondered if I would be able to suction her, and if I would even know when to try to help her breathe more easily. I was scared and nervously prayerful as I carefully slid in next to her fragile, warm body.

After the first time I removed the congestion from Cameron's throat, I felt myself relax. I even felt I could try to sing the song we used to share in the first months of her life: a made-up lullaby about protective "swooping angels, winging high, swinging low." There was a pattern of house sounds that came and went throughout night. Every few hours we could hear the hungry newborn cry and Blyth would tiptoe past Cameron's room to feed Eliza. Taylor always seemed to manage to sleep through these nights. The early mornings were quiet, with all outdoor sounds muffled by the snow on the ground.

One morning, though, we woke up to the clunk and scrape of snow shovels, the occasional plow passing on our dead-end street, and the delighted squeals of children building snowmen instead of going to school. The Boston blizzard of 2001 had arrived. In the house in Newton, the swirling weather was a formidable background for the crisis of Cameron's first bout of pneumonia.

I went with Blyth to take Cameron to the doctor, where she was officially diagnosed with pneumonia. Afterward, we went to the hospital for an x-ray to confirm the illness, so often fatal to infants with Tay Sachs. Dr. Goldstein gave Cameron two shots in her thigh muscles and said she would be better in about two days.

In fact, it took Cameron five days to regain the strength she needed to eat her soft food. She was too exhausted even to use her special slow-release bottle, designed for babies who have lost their swallowing reflex. We all felt the anxiety of the struggle to help the little one swallow her daily medications and essential antibiotics. Cameron did not smile for five days. She developed black circles under her beautiful blue eyes, stains that were dramatic against her porcelain skin. These days forced us all, but especially Charlie and Blyth, to confront the inevitable end. How many more times would they be willing to have Cameron suffer through these medical interventions?

After Cameron got better, the nights with her seemed ever more precious and mystical. It was transformative to be in bed with her, breathing with her every breath, learning to follow her lead and to make the best decisions about her comfort: whether to suction, or turn her over, or to let her work through the breathing on her own. These moments in the quiet dark of the night were the times when Cameron gave me her peace, when the happiness came seeping through the sadness. And then we would both go back to sleep.

In the car on the way back to Washington, Grandfather Charlie and I had plenty of time to think about the contrasts that filled our lives during those days. They were times when we both felt overtaken by exhaustion laced with coursing energy, when we felt deep-rooted sadness ingrown with joy. In her ebbing life, Cameron brought us all the gifts of creation. This is how Reverend Eleanor Panasevich later described Cameron's presence in our lives:

> *Cameron gave us all a window into heaven. It was as if she had been sent by God to teach us the importance of love…. Love does not prevent pain or grief. But love will and does sustain us through it. And it is love that makes healing possible. …The two greatest mysteries we encounter in life are incarnation and death. It is incomprehensible that they should occur so closely together. Yet I believe those are the times when God is closest. Those are the times when we find ourselves on Jacob's ladder.*

ALIVE IN THE DARK TIME

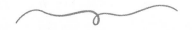

IT IS ONLY IN RECENT YEARS THAT WE HAVE TAKEN TO CALLING Cameron's father, Charlie, "The Buddhist-Episco," though it was years ago, during Cameron's last months of life, that he taught himself to meditate and began reading deeply in the works of Thich Nhat Hanh and other spiritual writers.

At the same time, Charlie and Blyth maintained a close connection with their beloved Episcopal minister, Ellie Panasavich. Ellie came to pray with Cameron and her parents every week. Once a week, they also saw their therapist and counselor, Laura Basili, who worked primarily with terminally ill children and their families. They continued to have sessions with Laura during the year after Cameron died.

Cameron's last months of life were guided by the mysteries of faith, which penetrated the days and nights of the people who lived in and visited the house at 21 Rochester Road. Cameron's father came to realize that as he phrased it, he "could know her and what she felt by holding her with a quiet heart and a quiet mind."

In this way, on Easter weekend of 2001, Charlie and Blyth took themselves and Cameron through and beyond a crisis. Cameron stopped eating and drinking on that weekend, giving the clear signal, in the way that all humans do at the end of their lives, that she was ready to die. On Good Friday, at St. Peter's Church, where Cameron had been christened a year and a half before, Charlie and Blyth and the delicate, quiet little girl meditated together. Titus, the new minister, sat with them.

Later, Charlie described what they experienced that night as they supported Cameron's tiny body, holding her stretched out across their laps. Both of Cameron's parents saw her appearance change as they sat in silence in the small chapel filled with flowers and mosses. Her father described that what they saw was a radiance reaching out from Cameron's pale body. He said to me on the phone, "All I could think of was Jesus."

On the morning of Easter Sunday, Charlie and Blyth woke up to the realization that Cameron would probably not eat or drink again without special help. They called one of the special nurses, Kelly, who had been present to care for Cameron during the previous months. Kelly, who lived in New Hampshire, told them that the temporary feeding tube (called an NG tube) could be inserted, if they wished, "to help her come back for a time."

When she got into her car that morning, to come back to Charlie, Blyth, Taylor, Eliza, and Cameron, Kelly did not know what their decision would be, but she wanted to be there with them if they decided to reverse the promise that they had made months before, not to take extreme measures to prolong Cameron's life. They had made this vow based on the fact that each time Cameron came back from a bout of pneumonia, her quality of life was reduced.

While they were waiting for Kelly to arrive from New Hampshire, Charlie and Blyth went up the stairs together and turned into Cameron's quiet, warm room to sit with her in order to, in Charlie's words, "meditate with her in the faith that we could find a path through this day." Their little girl was lying on her double bed covered with a soft beige blanket just the length of her body, which had been knitted for her by a friend. The soft lights that were strung over her bed were probably lit, and there must have been candles glowing on the bureau and tables in the room. The figures on the mobile hanging over Cameron's bed would have been dancing gently in the air. Next to Cameron's bed there was (and still is twelve years later) a photograph of the moon over a mountain in Tibet, taken by one of her godfathers. In a darkened sky, the moon shines and the mountain is grey. The only colors come from the blue, yellow, green, and red prayer flags waving in the snowy landscape.

Here is how Cameron's father described that morning when he and Blyth sat with Cameron:

> *After a time of breathing quietly together, I asked Blyth what she had felt and thought. She said: "I kept hearing the words, 'There are no wrong answers.'" I smiled at*

Cameron and said to both of them, "Those are the same words I heard." Both of us felt completely at peace with our decision, and realized at the core of our being that Cameron had told us she was ready to go, but that she would stay with us for a time if we wanted her to stay. Neither of us felt prepared to say goodbye to her, so we asked her to come back one more time.

We promised her that day that the next time she asked us to leave we would let her go. As the days unfolded, Blyth and I realized that we had been looking forward to her second birthday party with her friends and family.
—CHARLES PRIOR LORD, "THE WISDOM AND TEACHINGS OF CAMERON PATTERSON LORD," DECEMBER 2001–JANUARY 2002

Charlie and Blyth never regretted their decision to have Kelly give Cameron a feeding tube, which she did as soon as she arrived at the house. The day after Easter, Cameron was better and began to eat again. There would, indeed, be a party filled with family and friends and songs and dances. It was to be a perfect celebration of a little girl's second birthday.

23

MAY 4, 2001

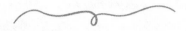

Every day brings more
Than the day before
Open any door
And say hello, hello, hello

It's the same bright sun
Shines on everyone
And though the clouds may come
Just say hello, hello, hello

Shalom, Hola, Ciao, Bonjour, Moshi moshi, Salaam,
Yo bo say, Neeha, Chesh
—DAN ZANES & FRIENDS, "HELLO," ROCKET SHIP BEACH

THIS WAS ONE OF THE SONGS THAT WAS OFTEN SUNG DURING
Cameron's last year. Her parents called it her "Happy Song."
We sang it when we danced in the garden at Cameron's

second birthday. It was a day that seemed to fulfill every dream for a child's second birthday. On a warm, shirt-sleeve afternoon, yellow and white daffodils were blooming around the edges of the grass.

In fact, it was such a lovely day that, had the pool been uncovered, we could even have gone swimming. It was a good thing, though, that the pool could not be used, because the backyard was brimming with toddling children and crawling babies who were safely able to run, scoot, play, and dance in the colorful fenced-in garden.

We had made oversized crepe paper flowers that were spotted about on the fence, chairs, and tree trunks. At the center of the party Cameron lay, transparently pale, on her makeshift throne: her blue beanbag seat covered with a white sheepskin throw, all set up high on a chair brought down from the living room. A huge purple, pink, and yellow flower sat high on a stick next to her. When she was not being carried in someone's arms, there was always someone near Cameron, holding her hand, touching the pressure points on her wrists, or stroking her chest—trying to still the small seizures that would shiver their way through her medication.

Along with the toddlers and babies, the scene in the garden included families and friends talking and laughing. Mothers were nursing their youngest ones. Fathers were holding their babies in packs so they could look out and become part of the celebration, with its motion of colors, music, and laughter. There were blue and green quilts scattered about the grass so that people could sit or sprawl as they listened and watched.

As I looked around, I could see Charlie and Tim holding our newest grandchildren, Annie and Eliza. Sometimes,
watching them, I could not tell which man was the father
and which the uncle. They looked so much alike at that time
in their lives. I remember Annie in a blue-smocked dress,
nine months old at the time, always crawling away off the
edges of the quilt and onto the grass, with father or uncle
reaching after her.

Scattered about the yard were tables covered with light
blue checkered tablecloths set up with food and drinks.
Another table held stickers, markers, and crayons so that anyone who wished could write a message to Cameron or make a
drawing for her. Nearby was a Polaroid camera so that a picture of the author could accompany the message. The two-,
three-, and four-year-olds had stools to stand on so that they
could be high enough at the table to bend over their creations.
And so they did, all afternoon, coming and going to embellish
their works. A large heavy piece of white cardboard was set up
behind Cameron which, at the end of the afternoon, was filled
with people's thoughts, memories, and pictures.

The day was reminiscent of Breughel's Children's
Games painting. Dan Zanes' lively band played almost con-
tinuously. The presence of Dan Zanes' group of four young
musicians was a gift from Miko and Deirdre, who knew
that Dan's music was Taylor's favorite. They played, at various times and in several combinations, a base, a violin, a
guitar, a ukulele, and a banjo.

Everyone danced: parents with parents, parents with
children, mothers and fathers holding babies and toddlers—

sometimes on their shoulders. Deirdre, the "under-five favorite," was almost always found holding hands with Taylor and a ring of children doing the hokey pokey. Cameron danced, too—in the arms of people taking turns holding her so that she could be part of the circle.

Those days, in my arms, Cameron felt like a delicate doll filled with feathers; but no mere doll could ever make one feel so blessed. No wonder it was more than one person who said that to hold her was "like holding a piece of heaven in your arms."

There was, of course, a cake—such a cake!—a yellow sheet cake with yellow icing, Blyth's "Cameron color." It was covered with candles and bordered with lush, baroque, yellow, blue, and turquoise roses. It said, "To Cameron With All Our Love." When her father put a little of the icing on her lips, Cameron's mouth opened like a baby bird's as she received this unfamiliar treat.

All through the afternoon, people were smiling and happy and celebrating this young life, just as Charlie and Blyth hoped they would. Occasionally I thought I saw a distant look in Blyth and Aliey's eyes, as they listened and watched. The last song that Dan Zanes and his musicians played was "Somewhere Over the Rainbow." Everyone knew the words, so we could try to sing this one. Tears replaced the smiles, as we sang what Charlie and Blyth always called "Cameron's Sad Song."

After this, people began to round up children and drift out of the yard. Long shadows fell across the garden as people said their goodbyes, stopping to lift up Cameron's delicate hand or to touch her pale cheek.

Grandfather Charlie and I had been staying at Blyth's parents' house nearby. Having hosted us so generously during these recent years, this would be the last visit for a while. While they went directly home after the party, we stayed to have a little supper and to be present for the children's bedtimes. Cameron's father read On the Day You Were Born, with little lights shining dimly over her bed and, as always, candles glowing on a table nearby. Charlie and Blyth noticed that she had a cough, but when we brushed her forehead with kisses, nobody seemed concerned. We went to bed that night at the Taylors' full of thanks for the gifts of peace and happiness that Cameron had given to everyone, and to her parents especially, who cared so deeply that she have a "real two-year-old's birthday."

The phone rang the next morning at 9:00 a.m. When I realized that it was Cameron's father, Charlie, my heart and head pounded. We were all on the phone listening as Charlie explained that Cameron had developed pneumonia during the night. Dr. Goldstein had come in the early hours of the morning ready to start the morphine regime, though he was also armed with a dose of antibiotics, in case Charlie and Blyth wanted to make her "well" again. Twice Charlie told us that he wanted us to be calm and that he and Blyth were at peace with the decision they had made to "let go" of their little girl.

24

SAYING GOODBYE: CAMERON'S LAST WEEK

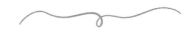

We need suffering in order to see the path.
. . . If we are afraid to touch our suffering
We will not be able to realize the path of
Peace, joy and liberation. Don't run away.
Touch your suffering and embrace it.
Make peace with it.

—THICH NHAT HANH

THIS IS THE PASSAGE I HAPPENED UPON ONE DAY DURING the last week of Cameron's life. Son Charlie had lent me his copy of Thich Nhat Hanh's Plum Village Chanting and Recitation Book. It was a profound sense of peace that settled in the house the week after Cameron's second birthday. People came and went, visiting for an hour or sometimes—if they had come a long way—spending the night on the pull-out couch downstairs.

Upstairs, where the family slept and where Cameron was resting on her big bed, often with her mother and father on either side of her, there was a murmuring quiet. To walk up the stairs to the second floor was to enter a different world, away from the workings of everyday life transpiring below. People came by with flowers and food throughout the days. In fact, there was so much food that we were having to throw things away (or try to give them away) before we had time to eat what people had brought the day before.

As we had in New York, when Hayden was in his last days of life, we took turns with Blyth's parents. One set would be at the house for dinner while the other family went out. The presence of Deirdre and Miko was an under-pinning of strength that week. They were taking care of details, some of which we never knew about until much later: funeral home plans, the search for beautiful con-tainers for the three divisions of Cameron's ashes (for each of Cameron's three burial places). She was to be partly in Green-Wood, near Hayden, partly at the Taylor family cemetery on the farm in Vermont, and partly in the singing stream which ripples around a special rock at the farm. It was a place where Cameron sat, cradled in the arms of her parents, on warm summer days.

Most of the time that week there were three nurses pres-ent in the house. These women were so kind and reliable, even staying beyond their allotted hours. In this way, the situation was very different from what it had been in New York, where finding people to help with Hayden had been so difficult and worrisome.

At night, before Taylor's bedtime, we danced. First Deirdre and Taylor would do a charmingly silly version of Swan Lake, which included elaborate "lifts" executed by Deirdre for a delighted Taylor. Our final entertainment was a circle dance, with Taylor pulling everyone together, gathering everyone from different places throughout the house. This, known as the "show me your movement" dance, ended with "put your bum in the middle." At this point, the circle would break open and extend into a conga line, which would then lead Taylor upstairs to bed. We sometimes carried little Cameron, ever so gently, at the edge of the circle, so that she, too, could be a part of the ritual. After Taylor's story, read by her mother or father, Blyth would do "the cuddle," stroking one of Taylor's arms until she drifted off to sleep.

In fact, it was Taylor we thought about most during those sadly beautiful days in May. What did she know? How could we make this week easier for her? What could we say that would help her let go of some of her feelings? At the birthday party the Saturday before, Taylor had been happily reunited with her friend Sophie. We noticed the two three-year-olds, face to small face, whispering and delighting in each other's company.

Charlie and Blyth had never actually said the word "death" to Taylor. After the birthday party, Blyth had a conversation with little Sophie:

Sophie: "Is Cameron sick?"
Blyth: "Yes."

Sophie: "Does she have what Hayden did?"
Blyth: "Yes."
Sophie: "Hayden died. Will Cameron die?"
Blyth: "Yes."

How wonderful it was to imagine Taylor able to tell the truth to little Sophie, though to this day, we are not exactly sure what transpired between the little girls. It was, for Taylor, too disturbing and difficult to acknowledge, much less to discuss with us.

On Monday, the day after Cameron's birthday, Taylor went to school as usual. She felt sick at school and actually threw up her breakfast. Someone brought her home right away. The next day, she wanted to go to school, so her father took her and went into the classroom and sat with her at the computer. Taylor looked up at her daddy, cried a little, and asked, "What will I do when you leave?" They went home then, and did not try school again that week.

All of Taylor's favorite people were in the house, wanting to be with her, read to her, and play games with her. Charlie and Blyth made time to be alone with Taylor every day, so that she could feel free to ask questions. But she really did not want to talk about her fears, or her awareness of the situation. She was reluctant to be in the room with Cameron all through that week.

Everyone in the house delighted in Taylor that week. We also clamored to be the ones to hold and feed three-month-old Eliza, who always had many arms waiting for her and many faces ready to charm forth her smiles of pleasure. At the same time, our thoughts and prayers were always with the little one in the big bed in the room at the top of the stairs.

For the first few days of the week, Cameron looked much as she had at her party. She was pale, frail, and delicate; her blond wisps of hair floated out onto the pillow around her sweet face. There were lights surrounding a soft, pastel, child-sized quilt that hung over the bed.

A few days after her birthday, I got to hold Cameron outside in a sun-drenched corner of the porch. I could listen to bird songs and, from her tender expression, I could imagine that she heard them, too. We sang the "swooping angel" song. Cameron's weightlessness made me think she might be able to float away.

On the 8th of May, Cameron's color began to change. The dark circles that we had seen with Hayden appeared under her eyes. Those lovely eyes—always so startlingly blue and shining—were greyer.

Cameron's breathing had stopped several times the day before she died. When Charlie and I went up to see her on the 9th of May—the day we were sure would be her last on this earth—she was lying in the big bed. Blyth and Charlie were lying on either side of her, both reading. I remember thinking that they were choosing words that they might want to have at Cameron's memorial service. The bible and a book by Thich Nhat Hanh were lying on the bed.

That afternoon, Deirdre and Miko took Taylor for a long walk and then to a video store to choose some films she might watch later, in case she tired of games and stories. They were thinking of distractions for her, so that, if

Cameron should die while Taylor was awake, she would not have to face the frightening reality of the undertakers and their somber arrival and departure.

Before Charlie and I went for a walk, we felt compelled to create a soft, blanketed place downstairs, near the back door, on top of the washer and the dryer, in case Cameron needed to be moved from her room before she was taken from the house. Afterward, Charlie and I went to the arboretum. We walked up and down the hills among the lilacs, which were of every color, from white to purple to violet of every hue, and in perfect bloom. The fragrance was dizzying. Every May thereafter, Blyth and Charlie would plant a lilac bush in the garden, to commemorate what came to be called, as renamed by a dear friend, "Cameron's Rebirth Day."

The Taylors invited all of us to dinner at their house that night, because Blyth and Charlie were so sure that these would be Cameron's last hours. Deirdre and Miko went home to the house at 21 Rochester Road when it was time for Taylor to go to bed.

When they arrived at the house, Taylor ran up the stairs and into Cameron's room for the first time that week. She blew a kiss to Cameron, limp and warm between her parents, and said, "I love you Cammie." Blyth left Cameron for a few moments and read Taylor a story, then tucked her in, checked on Eliza in her crib, and went back to her place next to Cameron. No one could believe that Cameron was still with us after the sessions of breathless quiet that Charlie and Blyth had seen that morning and the day before.

It was only about an hour later that Cameron took her last breath. Blyth and Charlie have always been sure that Cameron was waiting to say goodbye to her sister. Charlie called her grandfather Charlie and me. We went back to the house and climbed the stairs to have one last moment with our grandchild. Our lips brushed her a kiss where she was, still on her bed, tiny, waxen, and beautiful, her eyes open and her slight body covered with a blanket.

To give her parents more time with Cameron alone, we went downstairs to the living room, where we found that Dr. Goldstein and the pain doctor had stayed on after they had performed their official duties. All three of the nurses remained until it was clear that there was no more that they could do. I have no memory of who was in the house, but do remember that we all had a strong glass of something together. Charlie and I were in the kitchen when we saw Tim cradling Cameron's little body down the stairs and out the back door, with Deirdre following him. The car and the undertakers were waiting outside in the starry May night.

The next morning was another glorious shirt-sleeve day. Taylor set the tone for the day when she woke up saying, "I wish we could have a picnic, and I want to play with Annie." So picnic we did, in a lovely spot by the Charles River. The family and friends who were there sat on blankets or stood in clusters, forming a ragged circle around a barely greening tree. Charlie played his guitar. I think he must have played Cameron's happy and sad songs. "Every day brings more than the day before."

We did not think about what was to happen the next week, or the week after that. Cameron's peace was still with us, and we were alive in those moments.

25

MAY 19, 2001:
TO CALL MYSELF BELOVED

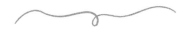

And did you get what
you wanted from this life, even so?
I did.
And what did you want?
To call myself beloved, to feel myself
beloved on the earth.

     —RAYMOND CARVER, "LATE FRAGMENT"

THESE WERE THE WORDS CHARLIE AND BLYTH CHOSE FOR THE
service of thanksgiving for Cameron, which took place on a
sunny, cold, Saturday in May, ten days after she died and only
nineteen months after she was christened in the same church.

At the baptism, the families had been huddled, facing
each other, in the choir pews at the front of the church. On
May 19th, all the pews were filled with family and friends,

spilling over even into the chapel at the back of the church. Along with the people who had been close to Cameron throughout her life, there were friends and relatives present who had not seen each other in years. Godparents and friends came from California, Ohio, Washington, and even from Scotland and Hong Kong.

Reverend Eleanor Panasevich led the service and spoke eloquently about the family she had not known before the baptism, but had grown to know so lovingly during the succeeding months.

After singing the hymn "Morning Has Broken" and reading in unison Psalm 21, there was a hush as the first of many people came forward to speak. A reverence for the occasion seemed to make the room come alive with a humming presence. A profound quiet settled during the readings and words spoken, though gentle reassuring laughter emerged when people mentioned the humorous moments they had spent with Cameron or Hayden.

During most of the service, Blyth, looking very thin but not exhausted and, in fact, radiant, held tiny Eliza in her arms. Taylor cuddled close between her parents or sat on her father's lap. Sitting in one of the front pews, I could hear the musical, non-disruptive sounds of children behind me, while I watched Taylor, directly across the aisle, head pushed forward, listening to every word that people were saying.

There were beautiful readings that morning. I read Jane Kenyon's poem "Let Evening Come." Grandfather Charlie read John Donne's lines that speak of ". . . one equal music. No fears . . ., no foes . . ., but an equal communion and identity.

No ends nor beginnings, but one equal eternity," words we read many nights during Cameron and Hayden's last months.

There seems no better way to capture the spirit of the day than to hear the words of the people present that morning. Here are some of the things people said:

> *I was supposed to help you on life's journey, dear Cameron, but it is you who has helped me. It is you who has brought me closer to God. You are forever my goddaughter and I am blessed for having you in my life.*
>
> —NOAH EMMERICH

From another godfather:

> *I don't have any children, my brother and sister don't have any children—this is something my parents remind us of during the holidays. I've never been a godfather before, so, when I was asked, I realized this presented some serious intimacy challenges. Cameron is a beautiful little girl, those great puffy, rosy cheeks, and spending time with her was always a pleasure. But I discovered a deeper connection. . . . Without ever speaking, she communicated loud and clear to me that things were all right. Ironically, this little girl was my source of strength. In her effortless way, she guided me from focusing on my own sense of loss and more on the joy of her life. How lucky she was to have Charlie and Blyth as her parents.*
>
> —TIM LEWIS

Deirdre said:

*For someone who did not speak in a traditional way,
Cameron was a gifted communicator. I sat with her in
my lap shortly after she was diagnosed withTay-Sachs.
All of a sudden, I felt the sadness of her coming struggle. I
did not want her to see me cry, so I put a pillow between
us. She was not fooled. She peeked around the pillow to
check on me, at once to comfort me and also to say, "Who
do you think I am, a baby or something?" I knew then
that there was nothing I could, or should, hide from her.
She understood. . . . Almost a year later she had grown
quieter, hadn't laughed recently, her smile was a little
more sly. She was living at a different pace. . . .
As Blyth stood up with Cameron to take her to bed,
Cameron burst forth with giggles and laughter. . . . It
was a treasured, miraculous moment. . . . And, in her
understanding, in giving joy and love, she changed the
way we perceived the world, the joy and the struggles.*

Tim said:

*Cameron: You and your cousin Hayden were not loud
children in the traditional sense of the word—like my
daughter Annie is now. But in your untraditional
loudness, you taught us how to listen—not only those
of us who were lucky enough to hold and read to you
and sing to you, but even those who maybe did not
know you so well. I reckon you taught us to listen as*

*well—to the joys of the simple things in life and how
lucky we are for the love we have. And for the people
in our lives. And for the things we read that all of a
sudden make so much sense to us.*

*On the morning Cameron died, one of Charlie's students
turned in a project she had done for his class—a book
of photographs and readings they had done in the class.
And because, Cameron, you and Hayden taught me to
listen, I was able to hear this:*

*"Keep me from going to sleep too soon—or if I sleep too
soon, come wake me up. Come whistling up the road,
stomp on the porch, bang on the door, make me get
get out of bed. Tell me the Northern lights are on and
make me look. Or tell me clouds are doing something
to the moon they have never done before and show me.
See that I see. . . . Tell me that waking is superb."*

*Cameron, you and Hayden, like a chorus of light
together, have shown us that waking is superb.*

(quoted lines from Annie Dillard's Pilgrim at Tinker Creek)

And Ellie Panasevich said these words:

*Two days before Cameron died, I was in the house
saying prayers with Cameron, Charlie, and Blyth, and
they told me that one of Cameron's godparents had said,*

as he sat holding Cameron in his arms, that it was like "holding a piece of heaven in his arms". . . . Many of you are familiar with the story of Jacob in the Old Testament. In it, he has a dream. He dreams of a great staircase, or ladder, reaching up to heaven with God's messengers going up and down carrying his commands. In the dream, God promises Jacob certain things. And then he says, "Wherever you go, Jacob, I shall be with you, and will bring you safely home again." I suspect for Noah, the godparent, holding Cameron in his arms was like being on Jacob's ladder. For, if anyone was ever a link between heaven and earth, it was Cameron.

Cameron gave all of us a window into heaven. I know now that God spoke these same words to Cameron. "Wherever you go, Cameron, I shall be with you, and will bring you safely home again." Cameron is safely home. . . . She is still with us, because her spirit lives on forever. Her spirit is the real part of her . . . that part of her will never die. It will live on in our lives for as long as we live. Cameron is with God. And because she is with God she is safe. She is all right. She is at peace.

Then Ellie said a blessing and asked for comfort for everyone whose hearts had been weighed down by grief. Her last words were familiar to many: "May the peace of the Lord be always with you." Everyone answered: "And also with you," and Ellie asked that everyone greet each other. There had never been a "passing of the peace" quite like this one.

Instead of turning to either side and shaking the hands of the people in the pews behind and in front of us, we all got up and moved around the church. We danced while we listened to a recording of "Hello," Cameron's favorite song.

It took a few minutes for quiet to return after the music stopped. But when Cameron's father got up to the pulpit and said, simply, "Hi", the hush returned. Here is what he said:

Blyth has made a beautiful video, but before we show it, we wanted to thank you ourselves for being here and for celebrating Cameron's gifts and helping us feel those gifts so strongly today.

Cameron: When you were less than 24 hours old, your mom was asleep, and you started to fuss in that plastic bassinette that they give you in Brigham and Women's Hospital. I picked you up and you looked me in the eyes, and I felt a surge run through me, and I thought: "You are trying to tell me something, and I hope that it is good."

About six months later, when we were waiting to hear whether you had Tay-Sachs or not, you woke up for the first and only time in your whole life at 11 o'clock at night. Your mother and I went to pick you up and you looked us in the eyes and we thought, each of us, as you gazed at us quietly, "She's trying to tell us something." And I thought to myself, "I hope that it is good."

I went to the Charles River the night we were going to get your diagnosis and read and watched the sunset. As the cherry blossoms bloomed inexplicably in late November, I held both terrible sadness in my heart at what I knew was coming, and an incredible joy at the beauty in this life. And you began for me that day a new life—a life that was fuller and deeper, a life that all of us who've known you have shared.

On the last day of your life, your mother and I spent the day with you in bed. I've been telling people that one of your last gifts is the reminder that it is important to spend the day in bed with someone you love as often as possible.

We watched the video. We saw Cameron in the pool. We saw her being held quietly during her last week. We saw her at her birthday parties. Afterward, Blyth spoke. These were her words:

It is, I am sure you are all thinking, a profound and beyond sad thing to have your child die. My sadness lies in how much I physically miss her smell, her face, her exquisite eyes, her soft beautiful hands, holding her supple body. In terms of the big picture of life, though, I am not sad. In fact, I have often in these past ten days, as well as over the course of the past eighteen months since her diagnosis, found myself experiencing something approximating ecstacy. This ecstacy comes from my

recognition of how blessed I have been to know, love,
and mother Cameron.

Within two days after her devastating diagnosis,
I realized Cameron was an angel come to deliver a
message to me, my family, and our circle. Suddenly,
the leaves on the trees were more vibrant in their hue,
laughter was sweeter, tears wetter, traffic irrelevant,
people more precious. . . .

Accepting her purpose and recognizing her purpose and
her power, I was prepared to give her back to God, from
whom I understood she had come and to whom she ulti-
mately belonged. We shared her, He and I. Cameron is
now happy and safe. She was happy and safe before, but
she is still happy and safe. She resides in my home and
can travel freely with us as Charlie and I and Taylor
and Eliza move about. . . . And now I promise, dear
Nugget, my sweet angel girl, to honor you: to look peo-
ple in the eye when talking to them, to really listen, as
your Uncle Tim said—to really be, to feel, and to live,
honestly. As you rose, you have lifted me up with you.
So, for all of this I am happy—truly, truly happy. May
all of you here also, please, please share this happiness. I
have not lost a child but rather gained a new life.

No more words needed to be said. We sat for a couple of
moments in quiet; there were tears certainly, but no sobbing,
no loud expressions of mourning. Music began to play. It was

lovely music, unfamiliar to most of us, but the lyrics were printed at the end of the program. So we sang:

> *Time has a different meaning now*
> *Since you found your scarlet wings*
> *Forever seems like yesterday*
> *But only angels know these things*
>
> *You are standing here beside me now*
> *As I watch the children play*
> *To those of us you left behind*
> *You are never far away*

—CINDY BULLENS, "AS LONG AS YOU LOVE";
COMPOSED BY THE ARTIST IN MEMORY OF HER DAUGHTER

26

GATHERED AT GREENWOOD FOR CAMERON

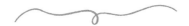

Laugh with me. Hold my hand.
We meet again at the source every moment.

—THICH NHAT HANH,
"THE CONTEMPLATION OF NO-COMING, NO-GOING"

THESE WORDS ARE CARVED ON A STONE NEAR STRONG JUT-
ting rocks that part the water midstream in a brook in Vermont. Wanting to know that Cameron's spirit was everywhere
in the world, especially in places that they loved, Charlie and
Blyth planned three distinct ceremonies for their little girl
during the weeks after she died.

The first of these took place only a few days after Cameron had gone. Only her most special people—her mother
and father, her two sisters, and Tanya, who had helped care

for her since birth—were present at the edge of the stream. It is a magical place where, even at the end of her life, she had been able to sense the flickering sun and shadow and the cool bubbling of the water. It is a lovely mossy, dappled place, the sort of unforgettable bit of nature which would remain in the mind forever, even if it wasn't familiar and beloved, as it is to the Taylor family and to all of us who love her. There, some of Cameron's ashes were scattered and swirled away in the dancing movement of the waters. This was the first and the most intimate of the three gatherings to remember Cameron.

The following week, the group expanded to include grandparents, aunts, uncles, and cousins. We were at Greenwood, where more of Cameron's ashes were placed in a grave only a few feet from Hayden. As we got out of the cars, Charlie and Blyth made sure that each of us carried a small white envelope, which we were instructed to hold gently as we walked up the little hill to the graves. The same people were gathered who had been together in January, this time not huddled and clutching each other to help keep out the cold, but holding hands in a circle on a cool and sunny spring day. This time, the grass was not frozen and grey but the yellow-green of spring; and the small evergreens, guarding the corners of the little plot where we stood, showed tips of new growth.

Once again, we spoke of Cameron and thanked her for the ways each one of us had been changed by her presence in our lives. For me, memories of those moments at Greenwood, and for the days after she died, are more visual than verbal: the barely blooming cherry tree leaning over Cameron's corner of the green space; the lonely drive home to Washington; the tear-stained face of a waitress at an inn in Connecticut, who cried when we told her the story of Cameron and Hayden; our tears as we read the letters we found waiting for us when we got home.

There was not one journal entry for that week before Cameron's memorial service. Cameron's death made me ache for both babies. Being away from the rest of the family, whose closeness was sustenance, left me drifting that week, wondering how I could help Charlie and Blyth through and beyond the grief that seemed so overwhelming, as it had in January for Tim and Alison.

At home in Newton that week, Charlie and Blyth were planning a beautiful memorial service for Cameron, which would be the last of her formal ceremonies, now spreading out beyond her immediate family to include friends who had played a part in her short, full life.

Charlie and Blyth had given a box for Cameron's second birthday by Cameron's godmother, Elizabeth, that would always be with them and, as Charlie wrote later, could contain mementos of her sisters' lives: "First ski lift ticket, feathers picked up on the Long Trail, Nantucket shells, Eliza's wedding invitation, and whatever else life might bring."

I am certain that among the things in this box must be quotes from a book called Hope for the Flowers, which Laura Basili had found and would read at Cameron's memorial service. It is the story of two caterpillars, one very young yellow one and one old. The young one finds the old grey one making a cocoon. The young one asks about this:

"Butterfly—that word. . . . Tell me, sir, what is a butterfly?"

"It is what you are meant to become. It flies with beautiful wings and joins the earth to heaven. It drinks only nectar from the flowers and carries the seeds of love from one flower to another. Without butterflies the world would soon have few flowers."

"How does one become a butterfly?"

"You must want to fly so much that you are willing to give up being a caterpillar."

"You mean to die?"

"Yes and no. . . . What looks like you will die but what is really you will still live. Life is changed but not taken away. Isn't that different than those who die without ever becoming butterflies? . . . Watch me. I'm making a cocoon. It looks like I'm hiding, I know, but a cocoon is no escape. It's an in-between house where the changes take place. . . . During the change, it will seem to you and to anyone that might peek that nothing is happening—but the butterfly is already becoming. . . . Once you are a butterfly you can really love—the kind of love that makes new life is better than all the hugging that caterpillars do."

The grey-haired caterpillar continued to cover himself with silky threads. As he wove the last bit around his head, he called, "You'll be a beautiful butterfly—we're all waiting for you."

At Cameron's memorial service at St. Peter's Laura Basili had added, "Fly free, Cameron. Fly free."

After we said our words at Cameron's grave, we found that each one of us had a monarch butterfly folded into the little white envelope we had been holding that morning. As we opened our envelopes the brilliant creatures lifted silently out and off into the air. They came out at different moments and seemed to gain strength as they emerged from the temporary cocoons where they had been. Some went straight up into the air and some landed on our shoulders and arms.

One stayed flattened, with wings outspread, on the small evergreen in the corner near Cameron's grave. As we walked down the hillock, I turned back and could see the winged orange spot still pinning its brightness on the tree. Cameron's father told me later that he hoped that some of these monarchs would spin cocoons every year near our little hill at Greenwood.

Each of the families went away with their children for several weeks after the burials. It happened that both families had friends who could provide places that were perfect for a "recovery" vacation. They hoped, I imagine, that they could live with the beautiful memories and leave behind some of the sadness of medications, doctors, and the intensity that had surrounded those last days—and, in fact, years.

AFTERWORD

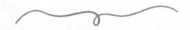

THIS BOOK WAS BASED ON A JOURNAL THAT I BEGAN IN 1997, the year that Taylor was born. The writing continued through the death of Cameron in May 2001.

The substance of the journal was given a more concrete form thanks to work done with four friends who rented a room at The Writer's Conference in Bethesda, Maryland. We met every two weeks for three years. Each of us was writing a memoir. I am forever indebted to the other four members of this group: Maureen Hinkle, John Malin, Bill Newlin, and Louisa Newlin, for their advice and suggestions, without which this would have been a very different creation.

We have lost our beloved patriarch, Grandfather Charlie, since I finished writing. He died in 2016.

We have gained two new family members: Mary Stinson Lord was born to Tim and Alison in 2005. Charles Anson Lord Wright was born to Deirdre and her partner, Alex Wright, in 2008. Tim was one of the first to visit

Deirdre and the new baby boy in the early morning after he was born. I saw Tim lean over the swaddled newborn to say some words that I, standing in the back of the room, could not hear. I did hear Deirdre's answer, though: "He has big shoes to fill."

Taylor will graduate from college in 2020. She's planning to go on to medical school to become a pediatrician. Annie and Eliza are seniors in two different high schools and will graduate in 2019. Mary is in sixth grade; her cousin and good friend Charlie is in fourth grade at the same school.

Blyth founded and manages a non-profit foundation, Courageous Parents Network, whose mission is "to empower parents of families living with serious illness." Charlie is a principal of Renew Energy Partners, an energy efficiency/clean on-site energy finance and development firm focusing on sustainable infrastructure (energy, waste, and water), with an emphasis on emerging markets.

Alison is an executive at Google in New York. Tim continues as co-founder and director of Dreamyard, the non-profit he and his partner Jason founded 25 years ago to "build pathways of equity and opportunity for youth in the Bronx." Dreamyard is now the largest arts organization in the Bronx.

Deirdre is an energy entrepreneur and runs a software-as-a-service business called the Megawatt Hour, which brings transparency and savings to commercial and industrial customers. She is also on the board of several renewable energy organizations.

Tim served as Board Chair of The National Tay-Sachs and Allied Diseases Foundation for several years after the babies died. When Hayden and Cameron were alive, they and the parents and grandparents attended all Conferences. Now Blyth attends in her capacity as Board Chair, where she is finishing a four year term in 2019.

ABOUT THE AUTHOR

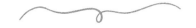

BORN GAY PATTERSON IN DAYTON, OHIO, IN 1935, GAY GRAD-
uated from Vassar College in 1957, majoring in Art History.
She went on to receive a masters degree at Harvard. She first
worked at the Decordova Museum in New York, in the cata-
logue department. After marriage to Charles Pillsbury Lord,
they travelled together to Panama, where identical twins
Tim and Charlie were born. For a brief time, Gay worked
at a small art museum in Panama. After Panama, Charles
became General Manager of Squibb in Guatemala, where
Deidre was born. Squibb called Charles to New York next,
where Gay became involved in environmental issues at an
institution called Consumer Action Now. It was in New
York where Charles decided to change careers, and they
made their next move to Toledo, Ohio, where they both
worked at The Maumee Valley School. Gay developed an Art
Histry course, team-taught with the Art teacher. From there,
Charles went on to head two more schools in Baltimore and

Washington. Gay taught at Sidwell Friends for eleven years. Finally, after living in New York for several years, a favorite city for both, they moved to a lovely retirement place in Westwood, Massachusetts.

ACKNOWLEDGMENTS

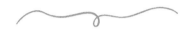

MY MOST HEART FELT WORDS OF THANKS GO TO HAYDEN'S
and Cameron's parents. The pain and grief will always be
a part of all of our lives, but especially theirs of course. Yet
they allowed me the chance to chronicle these tragic times
as their father and I experienced them. I did this, not only
because I love and admire our children, but I felt strongly
that others who were bearing similar burdens could benefit
strongly from watching the dynamic struggles and interac-
tions between these young families. In their journeys they
sought, found, and followed the paths which they felt would
bring the most peace and comfort to the two babies.

While this book focuses on the Lord family, The Taylor
and Smith families suffered the same anguish, as they helped
their children and grandchildren. They were all present and
involved in the babies lives. Peter, Anne, Tenney and Todd
Smith, and Jim, Lyn, Brittain and Elizabeth Taylor, were
tremendous sources of love and support Each will know the
singular sort of support he or she played.

I thank William Newlin, Jr., a publisher himself, for advice and encouragement to finish this manuscript. I also thank William Henry, a new friend, who also read chapters and encouraged me to move forward. I also thank Taylor and Eliza Lord for technical help and Blyth and Aliey for finding and providing photographs for the book. Blyth also read and critiqued certain passages and scientific facts.

Leah Gordon, the editor, and the designer, Domini Dragoone, each gave me help beyond the norm of their expected responsibilities.

And I thank my friends, for always being encouraging and present. Of course I will always be grateful to Julia Ogilvy and Joan Kavanaugh for their lovely words.

CPSIA information can be obtained
at www.ICGtesting.com
Printed in the USA
FSHW011830140419
57243FS